eHealth 2003

This project was co-financed by the EFRE fund of the EU and the Free State of Saxony. Responsibility for the contents of this publication lies with the authors.

eHealth 2003 Congress was arranged as a joint effort of the following organizations:

Bundesministerium für Gesundheit und Soziale Sicherung

Freistaat Sachsen
Staatsministerium für Wirtschaft und Arbeit
Staatsministerium für Soziales

GVG

ATG Aktionsforum Telematik im Gesundheitswesen

Schriftenreihe der GVG

Band 37: *gesundheitsziele.de*
Gesundheitsziele für Deutschland: Entwicklung, Ausrichtung, Konzepte
Köln, 2002 - ISBN 3-89838-029-7

Band 38: eHealth 2002 - Telematik im Gesundheitswesen
Dokumentation zum nationalen und internationalen Kongress
5. bis 7. März 2002 im Maritim Hotel Bonn
Köln, 2002 - ISBN 3-89838-031-9

Band 39: Sozialpolitische Beratung in Osteuropa
Einblicke in die Beratungspraxis am Beispiel des TACIS-Projektes "Governance of Social Security"
Köln, 2003 - ISBN 3-89838-039-4

Band 40: Social Protection in the Candidate Countries
Country Studies Estonia, Latvia, Lithuania
Köln, 2003 - ISBN 3-89838-042-2

Band 41: Social Protection in the Candidate Countries
Country Studies Czech Republik, Slovak Republic, Poland
Köln, 2003 - ISBN 3-89838-043-2

Band 42: Social Protection in the Candidate Countries
Country Studies Bulgaria, Hungary, Romania, Slovenia
Köln, 2003 - ISBN 3-89838-044-0

Band 43: Social Protection in the Candidate Countries
Country Studies Cyprus, Malta, Turkey
Köln, 2003 - ISBN 3-89838-045-9

Band 44: Offene Methode der Koordinierung im Gesundheitswesen
Zuschauen oder Gestalten? Strategien für eine Europäische Gesundheitspolitik von Bund, Ländern und Selbstverwaltung
Köln, 2004 - ISBN 3-89838-052-1

Band 45: eHealth 2003 – Telematik im Gesundheitswesen
Dokumentation zum nationalen und internationalen Kongress
21. bis 23. Oktober 2003 im Hilton Hotel Dresden
Köln, 2004 - ISBN 3-89838-054-8

Ältere Publikationen sind nachgewiesen unter: www.gvg-koeln.de

Gesellschaft für Versicherungswissenschaft
und –gestaltung e.V. (GVG) (Hrsg.)

eHealth 2003
Telematics in Health Care

Networked Health Care II: National Strategies – European Convergence

**Proceedings of the International Section
of the National and International Congress
21 – 23 October 2003
Hilton Hotel Dresden, Germany**

AKA

Bibliographic information published by *Die Deutsche Bibliothek*

Die Deutsche Bibliothek lists this publication in the *Deutsche Nationalbibliografie*; detailed bibliographic data is available on the Internet at http://dnb.ddb.de

Publisher: Akademische Verlagsgesellschaft Aka GmbH, Berlin

Copy editing and typesetting: Maria Zens, Bonn
Printing and Binding: Hundt Druck GmbH, Cologne

ISBN 3-89838-056-4 (Aka)
ISBN 1-58603-437-5 (IOS Press)

Preface

The national and international Congress *eHealth 2003 – Telematics in Health Care* which took place at the Dresden Hilton Hotel from 21st to 23rd October 2003 was dedicated to *Networked Health Care.* It was a milestone on the way to a health care system which is broadly supported by telematics and, thus, designed to enhance the quality of health care for the patients, to improve the data basis for decision-making processes and to allocate financial and personnel resources more efficiently.

The congress was organized as a joint effort of the Federal Ministry for Health and Social Security (BMGS), the Association for Social Security Policy and Research (GVG), the Saxony State Ministries for Social Affairs as well as for Economics and Labour, and the Action Forum on Health Telematics (ATG), which ist the platform for all the contracting partners in the German health care system.

The major section, which is comprehensively documented in this publication, was dedicated to the European perspective of health telematics. This focus on Europe reflects the coercive need for co-operation and co-ordination in this field. Experts from various European Member States and Newly Associated States presented their national strategies and implementation plans. They also offered insights into already-in-use technologies and applications. High-level representatives from the European Commission and the European health telematics platform EHTEL advocated the European cause.

Lectures and panels went beyond the national experience and discussed: What are the different stages of development? What can we learn from one another? How can common ICT standards and interoperability be achieved on a European level? What are the national prerequisites for co-ordination? How can contravening action been reduced? What are the legal, political, economic and social aspects of European solutions in health telematics?

These proceedings impressively demonstrate the necessity of political and adminsitrative co-ordinating action, they show the options for a co-operative development, merging the structural impetus of national plans and practices into a common European perspective. With our Congress *eHealth 2005,* which will take place in Munich in spring 2005, we offer the opportunity to record progress and to co-design the next steps.

Dr. Herbert Rische
Chairman GVG

Dr. Manfred Zipperer
Chairman ATG

Jürgen Dolle, GVG
Co-ordinator ATG

Contents

Manfred Zipperer
Introduction 7

Ole Henriksen
The Role of the European Commission on the Way to Compatible and Interoperable Health Care Systems in Europe 9

Otto Rienhoff
What We Expect from the European Commission 13

Michèle Thonnet
EHTEL – Consensus Platform in Europe: Possibilities and Limitations 19

Jana Zvárová
What Do the Candidate Countries Expect from the European Union? 29

Gottfried Dietzel
The Report of the Telematics Working Group to the High Level Committee on Health and German Expectations Regarding the Future Co-operation in the European Union 35

Panel Discussion I

Is National Activism Compatible with the Required European Spirit? 39

Co-operation and Convergence: Perspectives for Europe

Angelo Rossi Mori
Co-operative Development of the Health Care Infostructure for Europe 53

National Strategies in Centralized and Federal State Systems

Germany: *Manfred Zipperer, Norbert Paland* 59

Hungary: *Ákos Moró* 62

Spain: *José Luis Monteagudo* 64

Sweden: *Mats Larson* 67

Slovenia: *Marjan Suselj* 72

Czech Republic: *Ivo Burger* 75

Panel Discussion II

National Strategies in Centralized and Federal States 81

Jean-Claude Healy
National Strategies as Structural Elements for a European Telematics Strategy 95

List of Authors 105
Organizing Comittee 106
Programme Committee 107
Contact Adresses *eHealth 2003* 109
Action Forum on Health Telematics (ATG) 111

Dr. Manfred Zipperer

Introduction

My name is Manfred Zipperer, I welcome you warmly as Chairman of the Action Forum for Telematics in Health Care which has organized this congress together with the Federal Ministry for Health and Social Security and with the Saxony State Ministries for Social Affairs as well as for Economics and Labour. I warmly greet you on the third day of our eHealth Congress 2003 which is dedicated to international issues. I specifically extend greetings to our foreign guests and I am happy to report that over 150 participants registered for this international day which shows how great the interest in this part of the event is.

There are few areas in health care in which international integration and international relations are so pronounced as in Health Telematics. This is also surely related to the fact that Health Telematics is characterized by a very strong and, in the truest sense of the word, borderless community. This community serves not only principally those speaking English, but also has taken many terms from the English language over into its own, national set of terms, such as the title of this congress, eHealth, which is a well-known term in German by now. The Action Forum for Telematics in Health Care, on behalf of which I speak to you as Chairman, took this international interweaving into account at an early stage. This means that the exchange of experiences is marked by the following of developments in other countries, especially concerning eHealth.

With great interest, the eHealth community in Germany follows developments in countries like Austria, Canada, France, Great Britain and the Netherlands and in the Scandanavian countries, to name but a few. We see that countries entering the EU like Hungary, Slovenia and the Czech Republic are increasingly looking into eHealth for organizing their health systems. Experiences, particularly those to be made and already made in member states of the European Union, have played an important role in the discussion regarding the building of a telematic infrastructure in Germany. Likewise, we also hope that our experiences and results can be used by our neighbours in the coming years for the introduction of an electronic health card and with the building of a telematic infrastructure.

Within this context, the European Union is of special importance. Although health services and with them eHealth are primarily national domains, eHealth can play a significant role in the simplification of the procedures of claims for services in other member states which is the original responsibility of the European Union. As such, the integration of the so-called European Certificate of Illness, the E111, into an electronic health card is necessary. Due to this, the expectations towards the EU Commission whose representative Mr. Ole Henriksen I warmly greet today, as the motor for European integration also regarding eHealth are very high. We will accordingly listen with interest to Mr. Henriksen, regarding which role the Commission is thinking of pursuing on the way to a compatible and interoperable health system in Europe. Professor Otto Rienhoff will then formulate expectations to the EU Commission.

The Action Forum for Telematics in Health Care, which has organized this congress, is a member of the organization which concerns itself with Health Telematics on a European level, the "European Health Telematics Association", EHTEL. As such, I am especially happy to welcome the President of EHTEL, Ms. Michèle Thonnet, who will present the possibilities and activities of this unique European congress platform. Allow me a personal comment: ATG is a member of EHTEL. I would be most happy if the report from Ms. Thonnet would wake interest in EHTEL membership in as many of our listeners as possible. Our view should also be directed towards the countries entering the EU which are very interested in eHealth. Professor Jana Zvárová will explain the expectations of entering countries from the perspective of the Czech Republic. And finally Dr. Gottfried Dietzel will report on the activities of the working group Telematics for the High Level Committee on Health in Brussels and he will put into concrete terms the German expectations.

For the second half of the morning, I invite you to a panel discussion with the challenging title: "Is national activism compatible with the required European spirit?" During the afternoon, we will deal with national strategies, not only with those for Germany, but also strategies from many European member countries. Prof. Jean-Claude Healy from the EU Commission will not only assume the moderation of this presentation, but also take stock afterwards. During the entire reflection, he will explain his understanding of national strategies as building blocks for an European telematics strategy and I am already very curious about the conclusions which he will draw the national strategies.

Today you will see an extensive offering of facts and positions. I wish you a successful, international day in the context of the eHealth Congress 2003 in Dresden and, when you have the time, an interesting, beautiful city awaits your visit.

Ole Henriksen

The Role of the European Commission on the Way to Compatible and Interoperable Health Care Systems in Europe

I am delighted to speak at this conference on the future role of the European Union in assisting the promotion of interoperable health care delivery systems. This crucial field is at the heart of our aspirations to encourage European citizens to take more control of their own lives and health, as well as to assist health professionals in delivering advice of the very highest quality. Clearly, the development of electronic tools for networking information is bringing together professionals working in a wide variety of health issues and settings to the benefit of citizens and patients.

First, let me give you a quick reminder of the new public health programme: This programme, which will replace our previous mostly disease-aid programme, started officially on January 1, 2003. It will spend 312 million Euros over the next 6 years in support of three main sets of activities. We have ambitious plans to develop a health information and knowledge system, building on a set of community health indicators being drawn up through projects founded on DLO health monitoring programme. This will be the basis for a wide ranging series of EU public health reports tackling eHealth issues in the community. Many of the themes will arise from the so-called third strand of the new public health programme, e.g. healthy nutrition, good housing, control of environmental pollution and, of course, exposure to tobacco.

This work will be useful to a number of potential audiences, including health professionals, and competent authorities in member states, European citizens and patients. In order to reach such a wide range of recipients, we are developing plans for a new health portal. This will provide the electronic support for information gathering, networking and dissemination plans. It will build on the information system the Commission already has in place, that is widely used. We see our new portal as a central point of reference for networking information generated elsewhere in national websites and also via national partners, especially the WHO and OACD. A good example is the early warning and response system for communicable diseases. This will be developed into a fully fledged rapid response facility to deal with emergent strands, the so-called second strand of the new public health programme. This includes work to counter the ever present threat of terrorist activity. This is a timely moment to be speaking of the importance of such a facility. Many of you will be aware of the daily updates over summer on SARS on the new Europa website which awoke great interest.

The commission has proposed the creation of a new sensor for communicable diseases to ensure the timely transfer of information between member states and other communicable diseases networks. In due course, we hope to associate other aspects for health information activities across the range of communicable and non-communicable diseases. As regards eHealth, we want to ensure, in the future, our public health work is properly co-ordinated with work of DG Information Society. It is a part of the EU Sixth Research Framework, reflecting the growing exchange of ideas and practical co-operation between the two directorates in general. One practical manifestation of its co-operation has been the health online actions of the eEurope Action Plans launched by DG Information Society in close collaboration with us. A key product of the health online traptor of eEurope 2002 was the development of a set of quality criteria for health-related websites. As a follow-up to this, we will be developing a joint action with DG Information Society to explore the possibility of developing European seals of approval for health-related websites. eEurope 2002 has given now way to eEurope 2004, which provides for further work, or the possible exchange of patient data between health professionals, building on the recent initiative of DG Employment to institute a Europe-wide health insurance card.

This brings me back to the theme of this talk. The legal competence in the field of health care delivery is, of course, limited under the terms of Article 152 of the Treaty of Amsterdam. Nonetheless, although this is principally an area of member state competence, it is also an area where we think we have an important role to play. The issue also has a wider importance to us, since we are increasingly confronted with questions related to patient mobility within the EU. Past projects have developed cross-border co-operation in health care delivery, particularly in the EU border regions. Regionally based organisations for health care, in some cases supported by regional telematics network, are already promoted as part of the EU regional development initiatives. Indeed, we are becoming increasingly aware of just how many co-operations take place between health institutions, working closely together, but on different sides of national borders. The issue of patient mobility is also now very firmly on the political agenda. The series of high-profile judgements at the European Court of Justice, starting with the Kohll and Decker cases in 1998, are serving to clarify the extent of the right of patients to receive reimbursement for health care provided in another member state. Reflecting the importance of patient mobility, the Commissioner for Consumer Protection and Health set up a High Level Committee on Patient Mobility, studying different aspects of cross-border patient care. The scene for our future work in this area – telematic support for patient mobility – has been set by the health telematics working group of our own high-level advisory committee, the High Level Committee on Health. A link to the report that was published is (http://Europa.eu.int/comm/health/phoverview/Documents/hlch health telematics final report en.pdf). It will be put on the homepage of this conference, and I strongly recommend that you go there and that you take a look. This advisory working group consisting of eHealth specialists was commissioned by the High Level Committee on Health to advise on key issues and appropriate policy prescriptions in health telematics, including the role that the EU could play in helping to address some of the outstanding issues. This report has pointed out exactly that the same issues that apply to the exchange of patient data supporting cross-border patient mobility apply to the development of interoperable telematic systems supporting continuity of patient care within a national health system. There needs to be agreement upon a common data set and common standards for quotifying and transferring patient data securely, upon computer systems, upon enhanced attention to international standards, upon the promotion of translation facilities between systems, and upon open source software which are able to transfer this information successfully.

This is why we included in our plan a requirement for an eHealth co-ordinating mechanism, a co-ordinating group responsible for pushing forward our policy initiatives in this area, designed to facilitate and enhance the process of standardisation and interoperability. We also included the future launch of a newsletter to provide a public platform for member states to communicate with each other on their experiences and initiatives in developing health telematic systems.

Prof. Dr. Otto Rienhoff

What We Expect from the European Commission

From BICEPS to today

Expectations towards the European Commission have to be based on the experiences of the last 10-15 years in health-telematics. The current situation is in some respect dramatic, because several countries in Europe – Germany, France, some Nordic countries – are far on their way to implement national solutions. No longer the huge European discussing circus with many projects seems to be relevant: Everyone is happy that we come to real solutions – even if they are based in the national systems. This situation has emerged because of economic pressure in the different member states; now they are on their way to national solutions – including IT. The question is, to what extent we can still bring them together to an interoperable European approach. If nothing happens within the next few months we are heading towards a situation in which it may become much more difficult to achieve European interoperability.

I am kind of proud that I have been a witness to this kind of development since the first phase of the European projects (BICEPS) originally directed by Niels Rossing, who is present in the audience. With the BICEPS programme we very early outlined the aims of the Sixth Framework Programme, but most of the projects have never moved away from dealing with demonstration solutions. The financial figures of the European programs seemed huge, but in relation to the national implementation costs, they have been in fact tiny.

Two years ago, for the Sixth Framework Programme, the European Commission had the idea of very big integrating projects, and I myself worked with the German Ministry of Research to try and utilise the new instrument of integrated projects to move towards real world implementations.

As you know, this has not happened; the implemented projects in the Sixth Framework Programme are again small projects. They do not have the power which was envisaged. So we have not reached really significant project sizes, most of the projects which have been selected present very nice demonstration cases, but will never reach a level which will be of relevance for national implementations.

Another point is that the sustainability of the systems is a key aspect for the national implementations. The question is whether systems pay off after five or ten years. The business case is central. And the business cases have not been analysed enough. In the present situation, we need a positive approach and we urgently need European attention to interlink the national solutions which are popping up now. The only chance now is to build on very tough system management and very tough interoperability management for the upcoming national solutions. Dreaming in European projects – as has been done over the last years – has no future.

What is or should be the function of the EHTEL organisation?

Many years ago, some colleagues were delighted with the wealth of information the European projects provided – generating new ideas, specifying solutions, working up nomenclature and standardisation issues. But there had never been a service to gather this information and offer it to other people. There was always the problem, that we lost our memory. The data were not available to other people who realised projects on a national or a regional level. EHTEL, the European Health Telematics Platform, was one of the ideas to build up such a memory. Unfortunately, some other projects have similar roles and compete with EHTEL. As a result, we face an unhealthy competition in this area and this makes it difficult for the industry to join such projects. It is essential to establish a strong momentum to get the various efforts together and bring them into a stable, sustainable state – if possible within EHTEL.

International comparisons

Let us have a look at successful international approaches. I have grouped them into DICOM/HL7, CEN/ISO, and Unified Medical Language/Snomed. All of these represent a kind of success story. And some have a little bit more success than others. What do we learn? The successful ones work for several years in a stable conditions by users and industry alike. DICOM originated from the biggest radiological organisation in North America, with a lot of money behind it, and a strong interest from industry as well as from users. Sometimes conflicting, they nevertheless made it into a long-term working process and came to specifications which are extremely valuable today. The same applies for HL7.

CEN and ISO represent different stories and show different ways to success. The ISO process is rooted in a combination of industrial activities, governmental activities and user activities. CEN demonstrates that if you just take money, and if you just perform top-down projects, you may be on the top from an intellectual point of view, but you may not have the funds and the influence to bring your ideas into practice in the end.

My last point concerns Unified Medical Language (UML) and Snomed. Snomed comes from the academic sector. As you know, Snomed has been in a difficult situation for about 15 years. But it is interesting that Snomed is now financially supported by the National Library of Medicine in the US by joining it with UML. This important issue relates for me to the most negative aspect of the European development: the European Union never financed a similar development in Europe. If Europe wants to compete with such US-projects in the field of semantics, work cannot be done solely on a project level. If we, and that is my key message after so many years in this project circus, cannot establish a European institution which is funded for a long time, which does not have a project character, but can pay and run projects by itself with their own funds, we will not be able to deliver results similar to what the National Library of Medicine has achived in the States.

The situation in the European member states is complicated as well. The DIMDI in Germany was nearly scraped. It still exists, but was focused on different aspects. And famous institutions in France suffered a similar fate. Europe is in fact very weak on this. The leading nation in Medical Informatics and in nomenclature as well as in many other aspects is the US – whether the Europeans like it or not. And there will be no change to this if we keep on playing around like we have done over the last years in our project circus.

National solutions are on their way

The situation is that the national governments move ahead and lead to national solutions. As good Europeans, we want these solutions to be at least interoperable. Therefore we need right now – and not in five years time – activities on the European level, transparency and documentation of what is going on in France, in Germany etc. We have to make the facts publicly available as quickly as possible, we must make use of the good intentions to find interoperable solutions on the European level even at this stage of development. But I think what we cannot do any more to try to find a generic European solution. The right moment for that would have been ten years ago. But if we still want to bring the national solutions together, we need a massive process for information and transparency of what is going on in Denmark, Sweden, Spain, Germany, France etc. Maybe this at least is the chance to change and to support communication between different stakeholders and actors and institutions in the national systems.

Proof of cost-efficiency

The final G8 conference 2000 in Berlin, with Jean-Claude Healy on top, drew a key conclusion that is absolutely true: We need to prove to our governments that IT solutions in health care pay off, save money, save lives. That is something to hold on and to prove that Health telematics, eHealth, Medical Informatics are not just tools, not just playgrounds.

In Berlin, there was also a consensus about a second principal problem: IT technology is moving very quickly, but the methods of technology assessment currently available were developed in the sixties and seventies and designed to focus on slowly moving big technology, like nuclear power technology. We are still lacking adequate technology assessment methodology to do the job for IT. It is ridiculous how little has been done in this field.

In December 2002, the Pan American Health Organisation asked me to write a paper about card systems world-wide. They had been trying to find business cases, but the number of useful papers calculating expenditures and returns was less then five. So I think we have to focus on evaluation of systems again. We have to prove that they pay. And let me say to the case of SaxTeleMed, which has been reported here two days ago: If you calculate a five percent benefit, that remains within the limits of the accuracy of measurement. That is no proof. It is a good start, not more than that.

Conclusions

What do we expect from the European Commission? Nothing we can achieve in one or two years. Proof of efficiency will take time, has to be funded, maybe nationally, maybe on the European level. The same is true for a central institution like the NLM. Another stream which we need calls for more interoperability activities. But we don't need any more demonstration projects.

We have to move from technology driven projects to interoperability solutions. Interoperability has to be a key point, a key result of any project. Another very good message for the European Commission regarding funding of health telematics is: Please stay firmly either on the research or on the implementation side of things, but stop switching between them.

The real implementations, the national ones, are on their way now – with huge amounts of money, billions. This is a totally different world than what has been going on the European level within the projects. Europe has to try to keep the national projects together. Now!

Michèle Thonnet

EHTEL – Consensus Platform in Europe: Chances and Limitations*

I am very pleased to be in Germany again. I was here last year for the international day that EHTEL co-organised with ATG, and it is a real pleasure to be with you. I will not speak regarding my position in the French Ministry of Health, but regarding my position as president of EHTEL, the European Health TELematics Association. I will first present what EHTEL is today. My second point will be about what is new in the different sectors, what is new in the health sector, and what is the new challenge for EHTEL. And I will also discuss about what kind of limitations we have as EHTEL, and what are our driving forces. And I will finish my presentation by giving you some idea about the way forward for EHTEL and all of us.

What about EHTEL? Otto Rienhoff already spoke about the possibility of having a consensus platform and the need for harmonisation. EHTEL was created at the end of 1999. We wanted to create a neutral and non-profit organisation dealing with health care, in which all the stakeholders could be represented. And now we want to promote the use of the eHealth telemedicine and telematic supported services for all persons in charge of.

What is our policy? It may be one of our limitations, but it is also one of our driving forces: we are a membership driven organisation. This is to say that I will not decide anything. The EHTEL members will decide what to do, when, and where, and this is a big issue. This is because we want to be a neutral place, and have a balanced representation of all the needs, all the ideas, between representatives of all categories of actors of the health sector. We have to deliver services to our members and to the community, and we want by using ICT to facilitate transparency, exchanges of information and data in order to achieve efficient and valuable use of telematics and e-health and to provide added value in the health sector. The aim of EHTEL is to implement a broad use of ICT, and a solution of daily services for cities and patients. The representative of DG SANCO already spoke about mobility, but it is not only patient mobility, but also citizen

* This is the transcription of an oral presentation made with a powerpoint diaporama.

mobility and the mobility of health care professionals. So if you want to put this on the agenda, we have to work hard to change this in real terms. We want to offer some substantial benefits to all our representatives and to all our members and the community, and therefore we want to offer services based on eHealth tools because we expect benefits from this. But, this means management in the long run, and we cannot do this once and then lean back. It is a long run course.

How do we deal with this? The present organisation of EHTEL is on a voluntary basis; members choose to work on some issues, we are organised in different actor groups (HC authorities; HC professionals; Patients, consumers, citizens representatives; HC insurers; Industry), but we also had some burning questions and installed task forces to tackle these special questions. We have set up a new initiative, the EHTEL-like-Organisation (ELO) to promote the EHTEL vision, the EHTEL problems, questions and solutions to other countries on the national level. In Denmark, in Finland, France and Germany, in Italy, in Spain, and Sweden already exist, but we need to work together to harmonise and interconnect these national platforms.

What are the challenges EHTEL has to face? They are based on this new environment which is generated by changes in the health sector and new businesses. What can we see in the new business? There are transformations in any sector, reflecting the evolving society. We observe a collapse of time and distance, there is a shift to a 'buyer' viewpoint. In the health sector, changes occur via health care professionals or hospitals, but also through insurance organisation as well as through new services to patients and citizens. It is a broad evolution. Workflows span multiple organisations so it is not so easy. One common feature for this new environment is that we have continued commoditization and price and margin erosion. So it is a big challenge. In conclusion the business evolution is accelerated. This is the reason why we need to be connected in order to be able to react very quickly.

In this new environment, there is also new evidence that we reached the end of the "Solow" Paradox. What is the Solow Paradox? It was in the US in the nineteennineties: Mr. Solow and every one who was in line with this declaration said that in all studies, in all projects, in all action in the US, we can see everywhere computers. But if you want to look at the statistics, and the return on the investment with computer, you don't see anything. It was the paradox of Solow. But now the new studies of 2001 and 2002 show that we can see a beginning of a link between the ICT development and the increase in GDP and in productivity. But it is not as obvious as other figures are. Why? Because these investments and the return on these investments are not yet visible. It is visible on your implementation plan, or on your "document of work" for the European projects because everyone has to write it. At the end of the day If you look under the real exploitation plans, you will not see many reproductible features. This is because the performance is not in the technology, and for the moment not in the implementation plan, but it lies in the integration of technology and of knowledge and organisation. A last point in this context is until now in most cases: The new systems build up have been evaluated by the people who built it. But we cannot go further like this. The new systems must be assessed by people who need it and will use this.

What about the health sector? There are a few points new to this, and I will outline two of them. The first is: the health sector differs strongly from others, because you can choose to buy a TV, you can choose to drive a car, you can choose to go on holidays abroad, but you cannot choose to be ill or not. The health sector concerns everyone, and thus a huge population is afflicted. The other points deal with the evolving society: there is a lack of ICT investment and increasing budget constraints, we have to face with an ageing population, as well as growing expectations from patients, from citizens and also from health care professionals. The DG SANCO representative already spoke about the high-level reflection process regarding patient mobility. But just referring back from our Maastricht Treaty, we all know that everyone is concerned and everyone has the right to be cared from everywhere with the same quality of services. The last, but may be most important specificity of the health care sector is the neceesity of trust. In no other important sector is so much confidence needed as in the health one.

We are used to deal in the health sector with all the discontentment I pointed out. But we also need to keep in mind another crucial aspect: the global importance of the health sector. In the economic arena the health sector is an important carrier, an important employment area, and we must not forget this when we want to go further. Now, if we combine those features, what does this mean for the health sector and ICT? A solution in this field will provide a key instrument for coping with European health care and social challenges because of the free movement of people. You don't know if you will be a patient in the future. So we have to confort our efforts on health and social challenge. And hopefully the use of ICT could give some benefits to the present inequalities that already exist in our countries. Also we think that ICT could have potential to be a significant stimulus to the European ICT industry in emerging global markets and to go beyond insular markets which are not very challenging for the industry at the moment.

I am sure you are all convinced that, in order to achieve better access and continuity of care, under the free movement of citizens, all around Europe, there is an obvious need for interoperability, because everyone is concerned, because a lot of data are to be exchanged. Health care and health are information intensive. We need to set up customized tools in order to allow the development of those exchanges. In order to gain these benefits from eHealth, we need to develop and structure coherent basic features like an interoperable infrastructure, but we also need an infostructure built upon this interoperable secure infrastructure. This can only be done if we share some common view all over Europe, some common priorities and coherent policies. If this is not the case, we will just be floating in the sea, and not be on board of the ship. If we want to be connected, if we want to pave the way of harmonisation, we need to build connectivity. And the problem is that we have so many diverse systems that it is very difficult to resolve this contradiction. We need to implement a minimum set of standards to permit a real connectivity, not only on the new projects just to display the results, but in the real world. This is not only infrastructure, but also infostructure we will have to deal with, at the different levels of intermediation services, included methodology tools (like UML for example) and semantic or medical classifications (ICD 10 or / and SNOMED), as well as identity and security issues. We have to have some common vision about the semantics, too. It is to take the present system and to try to change it, to have business cases, and not to say we stop now, we want to have a new project, we want to rebuild new things. No – we have it. Now we need to go forward with this system.

How to go forward? We need a lot of communication and for this we need to have all the people involved, present and active at the same table, not only the architects but also the users; we need to have such a neutral forum with all the stakeholders. And that is one of the reasons why we think that EHTEL could be a good way to do this. But if you put everyone around the table, you will get as many ideas as you people present. The process becomes very difficult and we have also to avoid to "over-specify" things. For example, in terms of already-in-use technologies regarding identification, security, structured exchanges … . We have to use the international or European already-in-use standards, even if they have been developed previously for another sector, if the users' requirements are the same. We have to limit ourselves to what is strictly necessary and specifie to the health sector. To reinvent the wheel (by re-specifying and re-developing everything for the health sector) is a danger that we don't always have in mind. And this is the reason why we need to be involved and contribute to this high level process. We must not forget that subsidiarity applies not only to the political level, but also to the technical one.

What about the limitations? I will confine myself to the limitations of EHTEL. There are certainly different levels of limitation. The first is a generic difficulty. Speaking about ICT, you always begin to speak about technology, but in the next step, some stakeholders find that it could be necessary to change or update some functionality. Then new requirements and functionalities draw to a necessary organisational evolution. In between, technical progress is running. These two processes are sometimes running in parallel, but sometimes diverge, because of the two diverse speed processes and different kind of actors involved. So we need to develop new competencies and expertises – not only from an interoperable point of view, but in the medical technical fields. We cannot easily find people who are very competent in these two areas as well as in organisational and management field. It is even more difficult to find people not only able to serve their regional or national positions, but also the enlarged process of the European community. We must not forget that we are here not just for our own position, but to foster the European success, for the benefit of each citizen.

That was a generic limitation. We also have limitations due to the EHTEL status. And we have also limitations due to national priorities. A limitation due to the EHTEL status obviously is that we are not an institutional body. We are working on a voluntary basis. This is a good thing; but on the other hand, you are restricted if you don't need to work on a mandatory basis. Just think about how you deal with it in your daily life. And it is difficult for another reason as well: when people from the same country sit around the table, discussion on the European level could emerge and result in national confrontation. There are also some differences due to the history and culture of each country, and it could be difficult for the others to understand the reason of the present national health situation and system. Finally at the national or sub-national level, Europe is obviously not the first priority, except for people who work full-time for Europe – at least, I hope so. But at a national level, or in your own country, the first priority is national and / or "regional" reorganisation and implementation. At the third level, we can organise some cross-border issues, some harmonisation on the European level. As you can see the options are not so obvious. But because of the treaty, the free movement of patients, citizens and other persons, it may not come out as a limitation but offer a chance for a way forwards.

Let me now speak about limitations due to the European environment, which are many. First, there are sometimes differences between what we heard about policy and what exists in the reality. Secondly Europeans are very interested if you offer an idea for a new directive. But if you want to handle things not with a directive, it is more or less not so easy. Europe is constantly reorganising itself. Let me give one example DG INFSO was dealing with R&D projects and eHealth applications. Now, the Sixth Framework Programme is dealing with research Integrated Projects (IP), and Networks of Excellence (NoE) but nothing more regarding eHealth applications and implementation supposed to be overtaken by DG SANCO. Maybe we will have this discussion this afternoon, no further comment on this for the moment.

Another important point is that health is a national prerogative. And probably this is the major point. In this area, Europe could only propose some help in order to support some co-ordination work at the European level. It is up to us to decide to go further, even if it is not easy, because we have national issues which come first.

These were the present limitations, but there are also new limitations as well as new potentialities and opportunities. This refers to the new European enlargement, the new constitution, and the open method of co-ordination. I am sure you know that in this new constitution there is little room for general interest services. That is really a pity. But we have had the opportunity e.g. in the European Health Policy Forum to propose a very important and very consensual view of what health should be in the future in this constitution. And it was very well received by the Commission, by the Parliament etc. But the conclusion for the moment doesn't succeed as a chapter. This is to remind you that there is no chapter at all about health in the new constitution. But, as you know, the intergovernmental conference is over, discussion on that is closed. We can hope that health could have a better place with this new instrument, the open method of co-ordination, in which you can do the work progressively with some states and go further. Maybe there is a potential there, we will see.

What can we do within EHTEL? EHTEL has some driving forces. I just mentioned that it is difficult to work on a voluntary basis, but it also means energy to "drive" a non-profit organisation, because it is a neutral forum in which you can discuss directly and openly, with all the members behind you – representing all kinds of actors involved in and concerned by health care. This is a very important force, because you will be able to be representative of a consequent part of the health community: At the beginning, when you don't know the other people present, it is difficult to work with them. But in the train of work, you realise that even if you may have different solutions according to history or to position, finally you all face the same problems. And when people know each other, you succeed in working together in the same way. Volunteers to contribute to the network's strength exist all around Europe. But it takes time Finally, EHTEL set up a reference frame and a neutral platform to the emerging ICT market.

What about other driving forces? I don't want to go through all the items presented on my powerpoint dias. You can read them. But the second point is, in my view, interesting. If you are dealing with an organisation at the European level, even if you cannot join in every international event, if you have a representative there, your point of view could be taken into account since we have complementary initiatives with others. And we also lobby our governments. Regarding my position in the French Ministry of Health (eHealth Department), I have to contribute to policy making as well as stimulating investments.

EHTEL is also member of different committees as, for example, the European Heath Policy Forum. There was a set of NGO's who wanted to organise themselves together in order to speak on the same voice, to go forward on the health sector on European level. I just remind you some elements about this health chapter we missed for the moment in the new Constitution, but we will re-do this in the near future, after this discussion in Rome. EHTEL was also involved in an eHealth conference in Brussels in May 2003 as well as in the quality eHealth website communication that you have already heard about We also co-operate with other EU projects. We already achieved some positive results with other organisations, which you could recognise at the European level. EHTEL is also involved in the eHealth Action Plan of eEurope 2005. Moreover, members of EHTEL, especially from the health care authorities representative group, were members of the High Level Committee on Health Telematics Group.

So, what are the perspectives? I think that we could stimulate the atmosphere for eHealth in Europe. How to do this? The way forward for ICT could be to advise communication in relationship management. But not in order to, as we have heard sometimes in the European corridor, create new standards, but rather to reduce the number of existing standards, especially the competing ones. We need to increase the use of already existing standards. Thus, we have to stop "over-specifying" standards. Health is a specific sector, but in some clearly defined cases, we should utilise those which already exist in other sectors – especially at the "low" infrastrucutre level. We have to model ICT into health care and not the opposite. eHealth is not only a technological issue; it will change management structures in health care by using ICT. Technology could be a good key to have more efficiency in health care. But for this, we need to go further, deeper – not technologically, but into the different kinds of managing and/or medical processes. This is possible only if we work on re-organisation and necessary skills. Let me point out again the Brussels eHealth inter-ministerial conference and exhibition. There was a ministerial declaration on the margin of the conference, and all participants consented with the declaration to have full exploitation of eHealth, but only if we can link it to the needs of different stakeholders. Many important persons were present, including 33 ministers or health and telecommunication state secretaries. And they all expressed their commitment to different features. Three important ones, not only for EHTEL, but for the health sector in general, are: They agreed to develop national and regional eHealth implementation plans, not only projects that stop when the founding is finished. They agreed to work together and to have the possibility to co-ordinate for this, and I will ask the Commission in the course of this conference how to deal concretely with this. And they agreed that there is not only the technological level to be covered, but also the appropriate measures to be taken to facilitate eHealth from various perspectives: commitment was expressed to encourage appropriate legislative, executive and financial measures to promote the adoption of eHealth. This is decisive because it is the first time that, on a political level, people agreed on this. But it is only the first step.

What is the EHTEL most important challenge? We want to propose a Migration's road map, to facilitate and accelerate the satisfaction of all those different health care actors and stakeholders. We also will propose to go on open issues and preconditions necessary in order to implement these national and regional eHealth implementation plans in order to be connected with the other countries. For this, we think that this open issue on recognition could be classified in some category and I suggest here three different ones. I don't want to go through them all, but the first is dealing with the end-user's view, the applicant's view. EHR means electronic health record. The second one is the European perimeter with the European insurance card, but I put it into brackets because we have a chance to discuss this later. If you want to deploy an application which could be harmonised on the European level, you need to have this second level, you need to install health as an issue on the political level. Because the ministers commit to this, we would have to work on the management and the possible incentives at each sector level. And finally, but only finally, the third level is dealing with technology. We need to organise coherently those three levels, not only one out of them. We propose guidelines to go into this direction on a national and regional level; because we think that ICT is the main lever of organisational transformation. It is possible only if we have funding for that. Money is not enough, but is a necessary condition to push the means, to reorganise the processes, to develop the products and to deploy the services. In reality we have to manage all the needs, in the whole strategic included the impacts, the feedback and degree of satisfaction of the If you don't get this final point, I think that we will miss it as well as pour real aim.

Prof. Dr. Jana Zvárová

What Do the Candidate Countries Expect from the European Union?

Thank you very much for your invitation, I am very pleased to have the opportunity to be here. I would like to inform you about the candidate countries and the expectations from the European Union. As you know, the candidate countries are following the so-called eEurope+ Activity Plan. The European Ministerial Conference held in Warsaw in May 2000 underlines the importance of complementary European Union political commitments by creating a Europe-wide action plan, the so-called eEurope+.

The candidate countries are Newly Associated States. I would only like to remind you that Newly Associated States are the following: Bulgaria, the Republic of Cyprus, Czech Republic, Estonia, Hungary, Latvia, Lithuania, Malta, Poland, Romania, Slovakia and Slovenia. Regarding the geographical placement of these countries, they are not only Europe's closest neighbours. In these Newly Associated States in the Europe Activity Plan, they are running special programs reflecting the objectives of the operational plan Europe+ in health care. Basic objectives in the information society for all are improvement, the access to and use of the Internet; they are investment in education and collecting knowledge required by people through the digital age.

What are the IT skills in some selected Newly Associated States? In the Czech Republic, which I know best about, at the end of the year 2003, about 30% of the population is using the Internet. However, one tenth of all Internet users are students, and more than half are less than 25 years old.

We are speaking in the European programme about e-accessibility in Newly Associated States. What does this mean? It is the basic assumption for the future application of eHealth; on the other hand, coming from the figures, we can see a local portion of PC-equipped households in the newly associated countries. For instance, 13% of the households in the Czech Republic are equipped with a PC. That means a low possibility to introduce the advanced concepts in health telematics to the Newly Associated States.

I would like to point out two directions concerning the Czech Republic and eHealth activities. In the Czech Republic, we run domestic online programs in the period of 2002-2003. It is part of the Action Realization Plan of the State Information Politics. It is designed to introduce new information and communication technologies in Czech health care.

We also introduced several legal issues which are important for the use of these technologies in the future. In 2001, the Czech Republic legalised the use of the electronic form of a patient record without the paper form, with a guaranteed electronic signature. There is also legislation being prepared that the provision of a time stamp will be obligatory. A Czech law from the year 2000 requires data protection. It serves the protection of sensitive personal data in patient records. The protection of sensitive personal data is necessary for an interaction of electronic health records into the Czech health care. We have the institute of publishing of personal data and it is now possible to collect personal patient data only in accordance with a law within the electronic health record of a health organisation and with the informed consent of the patient. The Institute for Protection of Personal Data has to be notified of the data structure and of the data collection.

In the National Health Information System (NHIS) which is a source for many health data bases and registers, health statistics etc. patient records are the most important sources of health data, and they are used – in an anonymous and aggregated form – by the National Health Information System. The National Health Information System collects and processes information about the health condition of citizens and about health institutions. The managing health register was established in 2001 as a special part of this national health information system for the registration and the monitoring of patients. They are providing information for Czech and international institutions in the context of legal issues, and these national health information systems provide information for health research – it is possible to use the information they gather.

From the national health registers, we have a selection of currently accessible registers. There e.g. are the national transplant register, the national cardiosurgical register, the national register of cardiovascular intervention, the national register of vascular interventions, the national register of articular substitutes, the national oncological register and others. The health online programme is an Internet information forum for health care; it includes the ranking of health information sources considering the quality of care and the ranking of selected Czech health care organisations, according to the evaluation of their web-pages.

In 2003 the Health Information Forum was established as the discussion portal on Czech health care. This activity is mainly coming from the Ministry of Health, but we also have activities coming from the Czech government. And I think that one very important activity of the Czech government is the national programme of research and development in the Czech republic. Based on the governmental decision, the proposal for the national programme of research and development was elaborated in the years 2000 and 200; the Czech government approved the proposal of the national programme of research and development in April 2003. The national programme of research and development in the Czech Republic was elaborated according to the project called "Foresight". Experts from all the fields of research, education and industry in the Czech Republic were gathered to work on it. The wide-spread research topics resulted from this interaction, and I myself was working in the panel on the "Information Society", and also collaborated with the panel on "Medicine and Health Care". We elaborated some key issues that were accepted and approved by all experts. These key topics for research are: (1) Medical information and knowledge-based systems including personal systems. (2) Electronic documentation in medical, social security and governmental systems. We can now apply for grants to support our research in these fields.

At the moment, we are trying to get support for the development of these fields from national funds, although we have first experiences with working with the European Commission programs and projects. Previous experiences of Newly Associated States in programs supporting European co-operation were related to e.g. PHARE, Copernicus, Tempus, COST and now RTD projects of the Fourth, Fifth and Sixth Framework Programs. These are very important experiences for us. Currently, the European project "PRO-ACCESS" is going on, which is co-ordinated by Poland. PRO-ACCESS aims to transfer modern concepts in health telematics to the Newly Associated States. There was a conference titled "eHealth in Common Europe" in Krakow in June 2003, and the proceedings of this conference form a part of this project. There was also a special focus workshop entitled "e-Health Business Opportunities in Newly Associated States" as a precedent for these workshops.

We are trying to think about our roles and our possibilities in the integration into the European research area. We can see many points that can be discussed in more detail, but, e.g., it is very important to promote the RTD potential, also that of the NAS, because the European area is now really enlarging. From the historical point of view, this part had been connected – also intellectually – with the member states of today very closely. I would only like to remind the ancient European universities: the university in Prague was established in 1348, the university of Krakow in 1364, and Budapest in 1367.

There are also some things based on knowledge and education. I think, for the integration into EU, it is very important to promote exploratory visits and grants first, the development of assistant networks, training for project managers, web pages and info databases, integration of economic and in particular industrial resources.

Networking – I think it is very important for us to have possibilities for twining and to link health centres in member states to networks of excellence in Europe, networking on national and regional levels, and also to revitalise those networks and co-operation on a European level. It was also said in the previous lectures that these projects elaborated much useful information which must not be forgotten; it is very good that EHTEL is promoting this area again.

For improving excellence, it is also important to co-operate on an academic level. I will inform you later in more detail about our university activities which train students on post-graduate and Ph. D. level which is part of the project with the European Union countries; we have already made good experiences with that. The exchange of research results is extremely important to realise things locally as it enables us to evaluate the situation adequately. Post-doctoral studies, European doctoral studies – I think that the Czech university is very strong in this field, but sometimes you would like to have a re-establishment of outstanding researchers in the countries of origin. We also have problems which are due to our unequal economic possibilities. Some of the best people are leaving the countries and we miss these people in our projects because they are working abroad.

In the year 2004, in April, we will start activities that were initiated by the very well-known International Medical Association which prepared its Working Conference in Prague. The subject of this conference will be: "Statistical Methodology in Bioinformatics and Clinical Trials". As you know the field of Bioinformatics is strongly growing, and there is an interesting European project on Bioinformatics which is co-ordinated by Spain; they prepared a white paper. We recently published a paper with all the key messages in a biomedical journal. Further, we will have a symposium on electronic health records, health care registers and telemedicine. Our centre, which as you know was also established with the support of the European project, will celebrate its tenth anniversary in 2004.

We started with educational projects, because we think that it is a very important part of our activities. The next one will be on computerized guidelines and protocols and how we are to make our society informationally aware in the field of medicine. The internationally joined meeting inspired us to add a workshop on "RTD Potential in Central and Eastern Europe for Building Information Society in Health Care". It will be held in Prague on April 15th. I am looking forward to contacts with others, with EHTEL, and with the other really very good organisations that contribute to building bridges between the NAS and the member states in the fields of research, education and health care. The workshop will focus on building European research areas and the expectations the NAS have towards research and the technological development co-operation in Europe.

I would be very pleased to meet some of you in Prague and to discuss these things with you. The priority of the topics there will be priority of our countries for the future on RTD activities on the European level, IT accessibility in NAS and CEE countries, RTD experience in NAS and CEE countries, the expectations that derive from our participation in the EU. We also would like to say something about our national research and how we can really bridge it with the European Union countries. We would be very pleased to have the opportunity to learn from your experiences and to establish solutions for a better future in a smooth process.

We also invite you to visit our web-address www.euromise2004.org.

Dr. Gottfried Dietzel

The Report of the Telematics Working Group to the High Level Committee on Health and German Expectations Regarding the Future Co-operation in the European Union

Dresden is a key city in informatics in Germany, and this is the first ATG conference in former East Germany, and I am very happy to welcome you here.

I want to show you in what way we see connections between the work which needs to be done on the European level and what we have to implement on a national level – our key project is, as you may know, the new German health card. One important tool of work was the report of the working group on telematics attached to the High Level Committee on Health. This report has to be seen in relationship to different European activities.

This report must be seen in connection to many different activities. It is not the key document on a European level, but a document which was finished in a particular context; within a span of 3 years, we sat together with various experts from European countries who, at the same time, represent bridge-heads to other European activities. As such, a portion of this working group, which was established at DG SANCO, were simultaneously members of the Working Group of the Information Societies Technology Programme of the DG Information Society. Many of us have also worked with the eEurope Action Plan 2002 which was decided upon in Feira in June 2000 and then was followed by the eEurope Action Plan 2005. Both emphasized the significance of common infrastructures and regional networks which are to be constructed in individual member states. Then, as a result of these actions plans, we also received commission documents regarding legal questions about eHealth on a European level. These documents, however, have also a great importance for national implementation as the European legal position is also compulsory on a national level. The Sixth Framework Programme, which is embedded in the developments of the past 15 years which Otto Rienhoff has already shown, is running parallel to this. I am happy, and want to particularly make mention of, that Niels Rossing is here amongst us today. He was one of the first European promoters and I have learned very much from him.

In addition to all of these considerations, we also achieved a point of action this year. Namely, we not only achieved the communication by the Commission for the introduction of a European Health Insurance Card, but we also had the national strength in June 2003 to already agree upon very concrete implementation resolutions. As such, we are suddenly much further along with the European insurance card than with many national projects. I also have to say that this arises while this card is so much more simple in its functionality than what we are nationally planning and also more simple than the state of knowledge in this area.

A true milestone on a European level is the communication of quality criteria for the assessment of websites which are related to health. To which standards profile did this expert report react? These requirements, which arise from the health systems of our countries, are to a large degree the same. We see chances for the improvement of the information situation of citizens, for the training of citizens as well as professionals in health systems. We see chances in seamless care – a patient's data accompany a treatment – and we see chances in the support systems for those practising their profession. This is also life-time learning.

In these domains, the current report sought to fit together existing knowledge and to define options for actions. What we can achieve in our countries can be expressed in the buzzwords of information society: health care, seamless care, shared care, tailored care, integrated care, mobile care, home hospitals, consumer-centred care. As a whole, this gives a totally new perspective for patients who can expect better and more economical treatment, hopefully with our help, in the next years.

A key application which must be prepared is surely the electronic Health Record (EHR). This is the cornerstone and connecting link between all of the institutions which must concern themselves with health services provision. In order to make this totality function and render it exchangeable within a national as well as within an international level, there are precautions needed for interoperability. This interoperability is integrated into a telematic infrastructure system where electronic signatures and coding mechanisms are important. On a European level, methods for this have been developed early when I think of the early regulations regarding signatures.

What are the individual areas of recommendation which are set down in the report? First of all, this is the emphasis on the joint organisation of projects which are accordingly prepared and for which the information society assumed a role very early and which communicated an orientation for national activities over the last years. We absolutely need an overview and orientation for the assessment of activities as we have over 300 project results on European and national levels. This area of health technology assessments is exceptionally important as assessment mechanisms will tie on. Whether we form European targets or not will show itself in the next years. In any case, we will follow this path.

However, we can only achieve the interoperable solutions about which we just spoke through organisational measures, concerted actions which bring us further. This will soon be discussed in our podium discussion. Independent from European activities, we need mechanisms and forums for exchange between countries. We had such a forum in practice in this telematics working group. We worked together for three years and we do not want to do without this any more. At this time though, we do not see how this could be continued. EHTEL is a possibility, but we also need an authorative forum within the European Commission. Within these public health programmes, a newsletter has been announced but I do not know if there is already a first issue published.

One of the key services are electronic prescriptions or medication management. For Germany, we calculated that we could save at least 1 billion Euros per year with this. This will be the key utilization of the new German health card. The problems which exist for the implementation of this application were not concealed, but discussed in the report. This applies as well to the construction of trust centres, the components of security systems and the identification of patients. For this, we have already established that there are specific things which we cannot fully discuss. There are a few areas where the developments in the countries are so controversial that one absolutely must undertake follow-up activities in order to come to a European resolution. We have only touched upon them. At the moment, we have differing solutions in Europe for unambiguous patient identification.

In Germany in the new health system modernisation law, we have achieved something for the first time. The law was just signed by the German Lower House and, with this, brought into force. We did not think it possible, but we all receive an unambiguous patient identification in Germany. §290 says that the future German health insurance number comes from the number of the insured and an unambiguous patient number, so that in the future on the European card the key is on it for an identification of the insurance and the insured himself and, in this manner, one can bring data together. Data protectors are behind this solution; this solution can, however, only be used within the area of health and not within other social areas. The field of agreeing upon the nomenclature has also been addressed. This is then the result of our activities and about the limitations I have just spoken.

Now I come to a judgement of what we have achieved or rather what we should have achieved, but did not achieve. We did not write this report for the Commission, instead wrote it for the High Level Committee on Health, affiliated to DG SANCO, and then especially for the Directorate of Public Health, and then particularly for the Unit for Health Promotion, Health Monitoring and Injury Prevention. This means that the focus of this DG also determined the report and the recommendations in certain respects. European knowledge doubles itself every two years. I show you the fifth edition, which just came out, and you can see how voluminous it is. Still, we do not have the energy to transform this knowledge into what Michèle Thonnet postulates as performance, to transfer knowledge into application, to make performance emerge from knowledge. This is still the task that lies before us and which we must discuss in the panel discussion.

As we had a Commission speaker from DG SANCO in the course of this congress today, we challenged the Commission. We also want to challenge Jean-Claude Healy with the panel discussion. He will have the concluding word.

I hope that in the course of today the energy will develop to connect both areas, to develop something European in a combination of national requirements and the knowledge that connects us all. I hope that the power will emerge to find solutions on a European level which the Commission must implement, and also the power to find that we are nationally responsible for: to prepare the connection and harmonisation so that we do not run the risk of losing interoperability and connections between our solutions. This is the success I wish today for all of us.

Panel Discussion I

Is National Activism Compatible with the Required European Spirit?

Ole Henriksen, European Commission, DG SANCO*; Prof. Dr. Otto Rienhoff,* Vice President of EHTEL*; Michèle Thonnet,* President of EHTEL; *Akos Moró,* Ministry of Health, Social and Family Affairs, Hungary*; Prof. Dr. Jana Zvárová,* EuroMISE Centre of Charles University and Academy of Sciences, Czech Republic*; Dr. Gottfried Dietzel,* Federal Ministry of Health and Social Security, Germany

Moderator: Dr. Manfred Zipperer, Chairman of the Action Forum on Health Telematics, Germany

Dr. Manfred Zipperer

I would like to invite you to start our discussion: "Is national activism compatible with the required European spirit?" I think a lot of material has been accumulated in the speeches which have been given this morning, and I think that there will be a lot of work to do on this podium. I will give Mr. Henriksen from the European Commission the first opportunity to explain something to us because he has not yet had the opportunity to do this. We intend a clear separation between this discussion and the second discussion organised and guided by Prof. Healy.

To start the discussion, let me ask as a warm-up question first of all an additional one: Health matters are, as has been mentioned, the responsibility of the member states according to the European treaty. And the question is: Are health telematics, as eHealth, not a part of this national responsibility? Shouldn't we affirm national solutions first, and then European collaboration? Or what is the priority, what is the sequence? May I first give you, Mr. Henriksen, the opportunity to make your statement?

Ole Henriksen

I think that most of the speeches we heard called for more action on European level, and especially from the European Commission. I think most of the – I wouldn't say frustration, but – concern about this is that eHealth is in many cases health care. And health care is by definition out of the treaty of the community. So, we are regulated by Article 152, and it says that health care is solely the responsibility of the member states – for financing, for organisation, for deciding how things are done. Then, on the other hand, we have this patient mobility process, and it is barred by some rulings by the European court. This means that, in health care policy, there is a European dimension or an EU dimension of it, but it does remain outside the treaty. Which is a bit strange for us. So it is difficult for us to organise this for the member states, to regulate it, or whatever we would like to call it because we haven't got the legal basis in the treaty. This means that if you really want us to regulate the area much more, you need to go to our ministers, and you need to go to your parliaments, and make them give us the responsibility or the possibility to regulate or co-ordinate in this field.

The European Commission regulates many things – we like to determine the sizes of cucumbers –, but in this field, we do not have the legal basis to act. Thus, we cannot determine the size and the implementation of a health card. Not in a normal process. There was a suggestion from EHTEL to do this through the process of open co-ordination. And that is exactly on our table, that is our process on patient mobility, and that is our way into health care. They will make a report, and I think it will come out on December 8th. I am not sure how public it will be. But one of the suggestions there is to take this process further in this open method of co-ordination. This is my initial statement on this.

Dr. Manfred Zipperer

Thank you very much. The method of open co-ordination is one new instrument which has been developed to be active on the European level in fields which are the responsibility of the member states. And I think this is a very wise way because I think the member states can give and feed into this process what they think is best, and I think they can feed it into a common direction. Therefore, I think this process of open co-ordination will have its fundamental importance for eHealth, too. But back again to the basic question of this discussion. We have a lot of national activism in Germany, Prof. Rienhoff. Do you make a lot of critical remarks? Do you think this national activism is compatible with the required European spirit?

Prof. Dr. Otto Rienhoff

I principally agree with what you just stated. The national activisms are coming up now because we have not been able to formulate general European solutions. Every member state needs to move ahead, every stakeholder has to move. The key problem is that eHealth is part of the general health system. When we approach eHealth we transform the health system and individual roles.

Health systems are deeply grounded in the cultural history of countries. We are now in a phase where national institutions fight for their traditional roles, and it may take quite some years to move ahead. I wonder whether the direction into which we move might lead to different health systems.

I would not expect that the European governments are coming together easily in the field of health care. At least, the Christian Democrats in Germany and their representatives are against a European harmonization – as far as I know. I see a long process in front of us.

But there is another open door: consumer services. I believe that some of the European health care systems are so much in stormy waters that the wind of change may come from the consumer side, the patient side and from the side of private health care services which, within the next ten years, will be forcing traditional organisations to move. Myself being a doctor, I personally believe that especially the role of the physicians will change. If they don't wake up, things will change very much to their disadvantage.

The EU has a chance to work and to co-ordinate in the field of consumer relations. One should go through this open door now. We should look into the private health care sector and should regulate, or as a European citizen I would much prefer the word facilitate, that European organisations find ways to serve citizens in the field of health. This means that we promote processes which put national health policies in the second role. This is kind of revolutionary. But I think that this is a way we should go.

Sometimes I look to Switzerland. Switzerland has been able to move the health care system very much by introducing private elements into it. And I sometimes believe that at least Germany needs this openness so that our traditional system, which is about a hundred years old, can change to the better.

I expect that the European Union has to move into health care now because of all the national activities. It should take the chance to facilitate co-operation among the member states focussing on the consumer view. There is a chance for interoperability of national solutions - if we act now. Harmonising future European eHealth systems might be too big a job to do; it would take years, while the national solutions are on their way being implemented in 2-3 years. But if the EU will focus on consumer health it may be able to moderate and facilitate the interoperability aspects of national technical solutions.

Dr. Manfred Zipperer

Thank you very much, Prof. Rienhoff. We have the curious situation in the European Union that the health field is nationally dominated. But on the other hand – regard the legislation for medical professionals and e-commerce which is important for drugs and medical devices – each national island of health is surrounded by a lot of ships, or smaller islands which are already integrated in the European legislation. My question to you, Michèle Thonnet, is: Do you think that this being surrounded by a lot of different islands which are already integrated in the European community – and I think eHealth is already one of these components – will this put pressure on the national islands? Your country is proud of its national tradition. It is eager to preserve it and to continue it as Germany does, too. Do you think that these supranational islands around the national islands of health will influence the further development of the system?

Michèle Thonnet

Thank you, Manfred, for the question. I would say that some persons would like to live on an island, but some others don't like to live or work on islands. So, it is a choice. It is just like you said before that eHealth is a part of general health. It depends whether you are optimistic or not. If you prefer to have the bottle half-empty of half-filled. I would say that, because we all live here in Europe, we "aspire", like or sometimes need to go abroad, not only for working, anticiped health problems or holiday reasons. And so it is not only a question of choice, but it is a question for governments to be able to respond to the needs of their citizens, workers, patients and health care professionals. And I would also say that even if, for political reasons or for national history reasons, some governments want to stand still, maybe they stand, but the sea will not move from around them and they will not swim longer into the future. The risk to be drowned increase progressively but surely. That is to say that maybe we don't need to catch this with directives, with new laws on security etc., because regulation is only part of the story. Maybe Europe likes to do such, but we all think in this community that because people have to work together, because we have to meet and to live and to speak – simply, we cannot have these isolated projects, these isolated systems.

Rather than moving islands, try to co-operate to build one, then as many bridges as possible. Maybe it is difficult for the European Union to catch all these eHealth needs and solutions. But I would just like to tell you an example. Last September, we had a bilateral health ministry council between Germany and France. And we agreed that even if our systems are very different, even if the culture is different, we keep in mind that we have the same problem. We need to use ICT to better organise accessibility and continuity of care. We agreed that we need to have a secure infrastructure using cards. And we decided to go further on a coherent and convergent direction France and Germany are not two "isolated" countries. It is the same for other European countries. And so, we might build from these two islands, a bigger one at first, then bigger islands, and then you have a new potential European country. I would prefer to follow this way of working instead of regulating everything; to think about how to go further in a bilateral, cross-border process supposed to be possibly expanded to other countries. I prefer that rather than a top-down approach promoting a new directive. And I would personally think that if people agree on this method, it will be most successful.

Dr. Manfred Zipperer

Thank you very much. Mr. Moró, you come from one of the Newly Associated States (NAS). There you are responsible for telematics, for electronic information – and I think Hungary has a lot of national activism in this field, too, as I know. How do you manage this to fit into the European spirit?

Ákos Moró

Thank you for the question. First of all, I would like to point to the harmonization of the health care system and the health care IT system. In my mind, the unified health care system, or the common health care system, is a very long process in the EU. It is a very interesting question on how we can harmonize the IT system into the European community. What we learned in the past years from the Community is that it has a leadership or a very high role in the legal regulation, in the legal frame, in the co-ordination of the project and the standardization. What we would like to accept from the EU is the legal frame and the co-ordination. In order to fulfil this programme, we started six or seven main projects. I would like to speak about these projects later in the course of our conference. Now I would only like to point out that the key element is interoperability. I think that it is a very important feature because there is no function without it – in the hospitals, between the hospitals and the local government, in an electronic form, of course, between the local government and the policy makers. Thus, the interoperability is crucial. A second question is how we can provide the information, based on the IT-solutions and on the Internet, to the citizens. That is the other major issue of our development process in Hungary. The third fundamental question is, how can we implement the digital signature and we need huge support for that. It is the basic functional element of the interoperability process. These are the three parts that will be done in the next years.

Dr. Manfred Zipperer

Thank you very much. Prof. Zvárová, you mentioned a lot of activities in the Czech Republic as far as health telematics are concerned. Have you got the feeling those who manage these new activities concentrate more on the national development in the Czech Republic, or do they look at what happens in Brussels or in Luxembourg or wherever in the European Union? Would they like to co-ordinate or move directly in this direction, or is there a genuine Czech approach to these questions?

Prof. Dr. Jana Zvárová

Thank you very much for this difficult question! When we were creating the key area for research concerning health care, we were very strongly considering the material that we had from the European Commission. So our activities base on the experience that we receive from different European projects. This is how we are trying to render the national activism compatible with the European Commission's direction because we want to work in the European research area.

On the other hand, I have to say that we have many special things to consider. One of them is language. You have to communicate with patients about their health care systems in their own language; you cannot speak with them in English. The first thing to consider is that we have to use our language. In the research area, I have also noticed that it is very difficult for us to use e.g. SNOMED and these systems because they are based on the English language. We have terrible problems with the Czech language when we, in our research, use tools that have been developed independently from our language because we ourselves are not able to do all this sort of thing that was done in English in the Czech language. We are not such a big country with many researches which provide all the specifications. We have many languages, and we have to consider that in health care we want to speak with patients in their own language.

The second thing I would like to say is that we were very happy that we could consider many things together with our European partners in our European projects. We learned about many experiences that had been made in the member countries. For example, when we put our own projects about the electronic health records to the test under our own conditions, we found the core of the development is very essential for us, but we also have many specific features that we have to consider. I would like to mention only one of them. For example, in our health care, we have the unique number for the identification of each person, of each citizen actually. This number reflects very easily the age and sex, so it is not the best one. But even so, it will change in future. But there are situations when identification – with guaranteed security – is good. For instance, in the evaluation for research purposes for patients; they come repeatedly and you don't know that this is the same person because identification is not possible etc. There are many questions around this; how to really shape the European identification of the patient in accordance with all laws and regulations, all security prerequisites and all the aspects of anonymity, but also keep the possibility to evaluate the information that is given by the data for other purposes.

As a third thing, I would like to point out how really important education is. Education has a good tradition in our countries. If you don't have educated people, you are not able to provide them with important information, you are not able to transmit these pieces of information. E-accessibility and education in the broad area of patients are very important to create a basis for the use of the new tools. For eHealth, it is also essential to support research in this field. I think that we do not always mean the same things when we are using the same words.

We still have to differentiate information and knowledge more clearly. We ourselves are doing some work in this field, and as a first result, it is necessary in this Community to arrive at clear concepts and a clear understanding of each other. There is a big variety of problems, but I think that Europe is on a good way because it is possible to improve health care and, at the same time, meet the individual characteristics of the various countries.

Dr. Manfred Zipperer

Thank you very much, Prof. Zvárová, for this colourful and very plausible information about the situation in your country and what you think about the theme. Mr. Dietzel: Are the national activities not the fundament on which the European system will be built on, or should we first construct the European eHealth infrastructure with suitable, appropriate applications, and then adapt our national solutions into this European framework?

Dr. Gottfried Dietzel

Maybe the truth lies in the middle. If we analyse the state of affairs of today, then we can quite happily report that health telematics has reached politics. My state secretary was here two days ago opening this conference, and he really praised the situation in Germany and said that we came to a breakthrough in 2003: We have joint telematic reports of all the health ministers in Germany, we have an agreement with the "Selbstverwaltung" in health care on the introduction of the new German Health card, and we have an agreement that we should all work on a telematic infrastructure as a basis for a future communication system in health care. We see this success, and we would not have reached this success in Germany if there had not been open actions. But you cannot develop nationally and then expect that there is an easy way to harmonise.

On the other hand, these German actions are based on European knowledge, on a knowledge that was developed by joint action. But what are the problems now or today? If I refer to what Michèle Thonnet was mentioning as pre-requisites of successful implementation, then there were three areas: applications and they are knowledge-oriented and this knowledge is international. But then, the second important matters were the legal framework, administration and financing. And of course, legal framework is national, and financing of health care is also national. Therefore, we cannot expect that we get European solutions emerging all by themselves. This was one of the results of our three-year discussion in our telematics group: That according to the legal situation in Europe, we have the national responsibility for health care, and then again in some areas we have the possibility of European directives. But all of us felt very strongly that there is a middle layer where we can achieve our national goals to the benefit of the patient only if what we are doing is harmonised on the European level. We discuss this as "common actions". This means actions which are not European, which are not national, but which are under a national responsibility and harmonise together.

Especially in this special field of health care for a common infrastructure in our countries which is workable, we cannot just rely on European court decisions, on mobility as a driving force. But before we are coming to such decisions, we should try what is possible for us. And this is the challenge to organisation, which is a common challenge to the European commission, a common challenge to DG SANCO, DG Information Society and DG Employment as the player which is not present in this room, but which is responsible for the European health insurance card. I don't know if you have seen the picture with Prodi and Diamantopoulos. On this card there was not written health insurance card – it said European health card. But what we have implemented this year was the European health insurance card. And we from Germany wouldn't have agreed to this solution if there had not been a migration strategy of developing this visible card to an electronic card and from a health insurance card to a health card including the European emergency data set. We have the strength and the power only if we can align.

You see this wave from the European visible card, not taking into account all the knowledge that is within DG Information Society, and not taking into account all the driving forces which should be within DG Sanco – it is a very poor solution. But on the other hand we have the feeling that in 2004 we have the opportunity to come to a common solution, electronically, future-oriented and to the benefit of our patients. But what can be the way? There is only one method, a way to organise this. One thing is that the national governments tend to take all the knowledge from the international projects and then use it in their own countries. The key players have a responsibility that this is done in an internationally-oriented way. So is my state secretary; we are sponsoring this conference because we want to have a European solution for Germany. Of course, this is not a question of a German solution that then will be presented abroad and, of course, it is not a question of Germany waiting until we have the European solutions. So we take the knowledge, but then we want to apply it together within an international community. The driving force behind the use of international knowledge is industry. Industry doesn't want to have national solutions. They want to have a broader market. They are in favour of a European standardization. But on the other hand, they do not have the power to enforce this.

EHTEL is a good place to develop – on the informal level of the EHTEL organisation – common solutions. But then we need the power and we need the agreements of governments and the European Commission to find a way to apply these solutions in this field. On the other hand, we need putting pressure and lobbying towards European solutions, implemented by the Commission, in national solutions. So, it is my hope that we get such concerted actions within industry.

In Germany, we have a good example. Industry first was in favour of proprietary solutions. But they have noticed that they cannot survive with those solutions. Therefore, a year ago, we asked industry to give us some common solution for the telematic architecture. Industry was able to co-operate involving 30 or 40 companies and on the 2nd of June 2003 they presented a voluminous paper to my minister with, of course, common European solutions for infrastructure.

This showed us the possibility. But we really need now a new organisation on the level among the governments and with the Commission. We have the plans for eEurope. But these plans do not have a driving force behind them. This is a nice paper, but we still need an implementation organisation. And I hope that maybe at the end of this day Jean-Claude Healy and you can give us a vision. You spoke mainly about the possibilities within the public health programme, but I think there is more. You have seen that there are many more issues where we have to find such a common organisation structure.

So these are my hopes and my expectations that we enter an iterative process to answer your question. We should not leave contact to common knowledge which has to be developed by universities, by industry. But then again, in completely new governmental action, we used mainly to act on a national basis. In Germany, we have a federal system so we have a lot to do to get alignment with the states and the federal government. And now we suddenly have a fourth layer of governmental co-operation. Of course this is difficult, but we really need it.

Dr. Manfred Zipperer

Thank you. Mr. Dietzel, for this very enthusiastic description of the situation. You were directly questioned, Mr. Henriksen. Do you share his expectations?

Ole Henriksen

As I pointed out earlier, I represent one of the sort of three main players in this and I can only speak on behalf of this player. If Jean-Claude Healy has anything to add, he shall of course. For our part, as I read the legal basis, as I read our possibilities, what we could do is invite the right people for a meeting and we could ask them if they would like to co-ordinate the implementation of such a conference on their own free will. That is not prohibited in the treaty, that is not prohibited by anybody. That is the thing we can do, and that is the service we can provide. Of course, we would like to do so very much. I also have the files on several of our data driven projects where we have more health care data and this kind of thing. So this is a personal interest of mine, too. Because if we have the same system, we can also use some of the data – maybe. But we cannot impose it. We cannot impose on anybody anything on this issue, at least not in DG SANCO. But I think we could try to work towards having such a meeting, having such a co-ordination, and that is definitely now on my agenda. I hope this answers your question.

Dr. Manfred Zipperer

Thank you very much. We heard about the forces of patients, the forces of industry, the forces of government by legislation, e.g. in Germany. But not only in Germany do they press on the development of eHealth. Does this development become effective in the first place on the national level, or do you think it also will on the European level? Michèle Thonnet, what do you think about this?

Michèle Thonnet

I think the pressure comes from the citizens. While citizens are living in one country, they often travel or move abroad. If we want to succeed, we have to open our eyes to the world around. And if you want to be happy in your life, you have to be happy in your private life and your professional life. The same applies here. If we want to succeed, we have to have a good national system; but this system cannot be good if you cross the border and find things easier, better, cheaper than in your country. Nevertheless, we need to build upon our system because this system exists. We can not just forget it and build new systems. And as you know, it is more difficult to transform than to start from scratch. That is the reason why we try to build on real basis and structure the different levels needed : define what must be achieved on the national level and/or on an international level. But the difficulty lies in-between: How do we harmonise a system with different national approaches to the needs of citizens on a European level? In my previous presentation, I introduced the fact that we didn't succeed in having a health chapter in the new constitution because the discussion on that is closed. But I personally believe in that new instrument I mentioned – the open method of co-ordination, but I am sure that we will discuss this in more detail this afternoon.

Bilateral work is good, but it is not enough because it is not sufficient to build a system between for example France and Germany – we have to build a system which is interoperable with other countries as well. In this perspective, the most efficient way is not always to set a new law at the national level, or a new directive. We need to work together, but for this we need two things: I thank DG SANCO for the kind offer of supporting a meeting. But I think we need more than logistic support. It is one step. But we also need people who want to work together, and this open method of co-ordination could be a good instrument. But it also be nice to obtain a clarification of the missions and tasks supposed to be respectively endorsed by DG SANCO, DG INFSO, DG Employment, and DG Enterprise. And it would be fine if this first step into an open method of co-ordination will be an open method of co-ordination between the different DGs of the European Union.

Dr. Manfred Zipperer

You mention the open method, or the method of open co-ordination, which has been already mentioned at the beginning of the discussion. This is the beginning of the way. Let me say it like this: it is the way of the European Commission, but, and my question goes to Prof. Rienhoff: Do you think that national authorities, national governments, national patients' associations and national industry should put more pressure on the European authorities, especially on the European Union, to bring forward the matter of eHealth?

Prof. Dr. Otto Rienhoff

My colleague called for putting eHealth on the agenda in the European Union. Having had the pleasure, to harmonise the first version of the health professional card between the French ministry, French organisations and German organisations with some of the people here in the room about seven or eight years ago, I totally agree with Michèle: An invitation for a European meeting is nice, but it is not solving anything. We have had enough projects for many years now: We know how things can be done and know the different options. If we want to move ahead, we have to act now. And this means not only to meet but to write specifications and to come to agreements with the national levels, because the funds are not coming from the EU but still from national resources. The European money is peanuts in comparison with the money which you need on the national level for eHealth solutions.

So, we need more working task-forces. From the experience with the health professional card in 1996, working together is possible – even if ISO and CEN concepts had to be remodelled at that time. It was even possible to harmonise developments on an international level. You may remember the G-8 meeting in Berlin, when our colleague from the cards-team arrived from a meeting overseas with the message that also the North-American groups had agreed. It was proved that it is possible to do something like this.

It was based on, how shall I say, nationally supported specialists. There were Ottfried Schäfer, Bruno Struif, and Jürgen Sembritzki from Germany, there were a few other people who held relevant positions in their country and who could decide we do it this or we do it that way. And there were equivalent French colleagues. They were all brought together, they had funds to work together for one or two years, to do the specifications and then to return to their governments. There were meetings between the governments to agree on the results. It did work out at the time. What we are doing now in Germany is still based on the experiences of that work. And the people are still there to do it again and to work for the second generation of international specifications.

I am very optimistic that we can do a lot to harmonize national developments in eHealth on a European or global level; that we can become interoperable – but not with more meetings and conferences etc., but with the European Commission helping to finance collaborative work between representatives of national health care systems to find interoperable solutions. That is the one side I mentioned, the political side, the patients' organisations via parliament is the second part. But we need both.

Dr. Manfred Zipperer

Thank you very much. This is sort of a middle way. The European Commission has its part of activity, and the national governments or the national initiatives have their part of activity. I think it is rather difficult to find the adequate solution to come together because we have very different cultures, even in eHealth, even in the particular governments and member countries, and associated states. Perhaps this afternoon we will hear more about the position of the European Commission and how they think the future development in the field of eHealth will go on. I think it is a very, very difficult process. We have a lot of work there, but sometimes the wind of engagement and enthusiasm and activities takes away this mass of work and we sometimes see the top of the mountain where we want to go. I hope that we will get a glance at this top of the mountain very often in these days. I thank you very much for this discussion.

Angelo Rossi Mori

Collaborative Development of the Health Care Infostructure for Europe

I work for HL7, PROREC and OSIRIS, which is an EHTEL-like organisation in Italy. I will present the developments of ICT in health care as a set of steps that are marking the evolution of ICT in health care. We are going from the isolated applications towards a global impact. I schematised that in five different steps. The first step is what I call the paleoHITic period, the "ancient" period of the Health Information Technology (HIT). In old times, we had isolated applications: local technical decisions, each point of service was deciding itself how to apply health informatics. Bilateral communication was made by ad hoc interfaces, not standards. Then we had the mesoHITic period with the communication between the applications. The decisions are still local, we have bilateral communication and we start looking at the international co-operation for the standards, e.g. DICOM, EDI, CEN, HL7, and some middleware appeared. Then we have the stage of the neoHITic period with ad hoc integration. All the cross-border organisation, multilateral communication, webservices, integration platforms, most regions, most countries are at this level.

The three of them, the paleoHITic, the mesoHITic and the neoHITic periods form an era of the "preliminary organisation", I call that the proto-taxic era.

There are many local decisions of increasing size. So in each hospital, in each facility, in each health care organisation the size of the decision is increasing up to cross-organisational decisions. Many independent local decision-makers were signing the contracts and were making the plans with individual histories and different priorities. In one and the same region, we have structures at different evolutionary stages, because each local facility goes independently across this process.

And now, at the end of the proto-taxic era we are realising that there are many events that announce that there is a revolution coming. In all the countries, or in many countries, we notice position papers, ad hoc meetings, that show that there is an increasing awareness within the health ICT community. We see projects trying to develop new ideas. We see that there is a change of attitude there

We see the white books with some countries more in advance. The white book in the UK was published in 1998. We also see that people are trying to develop a shared vision and we see that governments are setting up agencies for co-ordination. Each agency is a national agency which often takes ten or twenty million Euros per year, like CIHI in Canada, for example. They produce basic reference material. And they produce an explicit strategy, like a road map.

All that is becoming slowly a reality in the "modern era". A new generation of standards is being prepared to face with this kind of era. And what is the difference to the years before? Action is now driven by political decisions. So, in most countries, in most regions, we have local decisions that grow up. At a certain moment there is an opportunity for political decisions that will bring the framework at a regional level, at a national level. So, we see the networks for continuity of care, the big data warehouses, the regional health networks, and the infrastructures. The regions are assisting the local decision-makers to make their job.

And then, somewhere in the future, in the "utopian era", we will have the "perfect" information society, in which the decisions will be taken within a national and an international scenario within a really European market, the global market. We will have real integration, local administrative organisation and clinical information with all the dangers and all the benefits of this kind of approach all over the sectors: health and social, but also environment and labour, and tourism – all the sectors of the society put together.

The eGovernment actions will be put to the extreme consequence. We live in a continuous process of change and adjustment. It is not possible to fix the evolution of ICT today. There is a continuous interaction between the new possibilities and opportunities deriving from ICT, and the new organisational models which are possible in health care. ICT is able to support the current organisational models, and new ones will emerge thanks to ICT.

At this point international co-operation on the infrastructure should hopefully take place. Why is it needed? It is an agreed fact that we need a lot of studies and technological assessment on ICT etc. I don't know if many banks and many aircraft companies made assessments of the benefits of information technologies, or how many studies were made on mobile phones to spread them in our lifes. Some things are so obvious they need no justification, anyhow. For example the chairperson of the US parliament for the sub-committee for health this summer was discussing the US act on the national health information infrastructure. The United States have private health care systems, which are yet in many cases linked with public systems, but they consider to develop a health information infrastructure lead by the government. In front of the parliament, she was telling that there is a cost of 5.4 billion a year for the repetition of tests, medical errors cost about 30 billion a year, and at present it takes 17 years for new knowledge generated by controlled clinical trials to be incorporated into practice.

All these topics could be assisted by health informatics – the proper health informatics. In Canada they made Infoway, and they are spending in steps, at the moment they arrive at 1.1 billion to foster and accelerate the development of the interoperable, Pan-Canadian health information system,. At the service points they have a lot of local systems, legacy systems inside their hospitals, and also in the private pharmacies, at family physicians etc., and they integrate all these systems through the access layer into a jurisdictional system. Each jurisdiction can implement the model in its own way, but with the local speed and the local constraints, so that the result is interoperable at the level of the country. Each jurisdiction will implement its own health information access layer to put together, to integrate the different systems. And there will be a registry of the people, a registry of the health professionals, there will be some kind of "domain repository" that is place for the images and the laboratory results. In addition there is something that is special. There will be an EHR repository, that is the one for clinical information, and then a data base for health surveillance at the level of jurisdiction.

And then of course they need a cross-jurisdictional "locator" for the EHR, because this service will be realised in different ways in each jurisdiction, and there is the need to understand where the patient's information is stored, when they work on the country level.

In England they already made a lot of progress, and with 50 million citizens and one million health professionals, two percent of the health budget goes into ICT, there are 20 000 ICT professionals across the country, 1000 ICT professionals at the national level, but they are searching for an acceleration programme. They realised that two percent is not enough; so they are going to four percent. I don't want to anticipate here the talk by Jeremy Thorpe. I just want to stress that in one country two percent is considered too low. They are going to four percent in three years. And this is a matter of 3.4 billion Euros in three years.

Kaiser Permanente in the US is a very good example, because they made their own cost-benefit analysis. They had a contract of four hundred million dollars in 1999. And they have made another contract now for 1.8 billion dollars for five years. This amount is nine percent of the budget. So, they will spend 2-3 percent per year of their budget to increase the really good information system that they have. And it is not a little organisation, it is an organisation assisting 8.4 million people. So it is bigger than many European countries, bigger than any Italian region etc. There is no profit, but they are not willing to lose money. They made careful calculations if this investment was correct or not. We are to learn from them about their reasons and to copy, just copy, their decisions.

We need to start a process of change management. Something that will never stop. When we start to enter in this evolutionary approach, we will discover that every year we need to reinvent everything, and that we need to follow the evolution. It is a matter of regulation, national and regional investments, observatories and surveys, education, standards, open source, open content, new organisational models, pilot implementations, incentives. All of that must to be put into the same framework, into the same vision. And what is most important is that the infrastructure, the public information infrastructure, has to be public – driven by the public, paid by the government, the national and regional government. The reference architecture, the content to be exchanged or shared (i.e. which data entries, which coding schemes), basic technical documentation, an interactive regional observatory has to be driven by the public system. This effort cannot be asked to be organized and payed by the local systems, the local authorities, the local hospitals, or the industries. It is a matter of governments, of authorities.

This is the opportunity for European co-operation and collaboration. I don't like the word 'open co-ordination', that is going on in Europe now. It perhaps will be the solution for us, but in my view collaboration rather means more freedom for the countries and the regions, too. To accept or not to accept co-ordination means something stronger.

It is not only to decide on the standards, that are already faced by the standardisation bodies. The big problem is to develop a common methodology to support strategies and to understand how to induce cultural and organisational changes. We should support the eCommunities and experts in health ICT to help them to meet, discuss and evaluate the solutions that are proposed. Thus, we are to encourage the involvement of professional societies in the clinical standards and we are to use the lesson learned to assure that innovation faces real problems and is always adapted to the local context. I have experience in CEN about this lack of dealing with real problem in the European standardisation bodies. I was one of the writers of the standards, but I recognise that we were far away from the real problems in CEN.

In the paper enclosed in your proceedings, I present some technical topics that can be faced through a collaborative effort at the European level. It is not a matter of treaties, it is a matter of common sense. We all will benefit if we work together in a certain number of topics. If we avoid the mistakes, we improve the benefits: the tools for large metadata registers, the tools for the large collection of clinical protocols, the standards on architecture, transactions, clinical entries, coding schemes, structured documents, the planning of a set of web-services to feed a series of portals, and the new organisational models. So it is something cultural, it is not about regulations. It is clear that regulations about health are not in the mandate for the European Commission, but to co-operate in the field of e-health is something that we can do without a treaty. It is only common sense to co-operate across the countries to avoid mistakes and to benefit from the other's experiences.

I call that the "AD HOC" programme of Advanced Development of Health care Content. We need this kind of collaborative initiative. In my view, we can start with ten to thirty million Euros p.a., it is not a huge amount, if compared with the benefits. It is just for installing collaboration structures, it is not to pay for the developments in each country; each country has to develop its own infrastructure with its agencies, its implementations. It is just designed to provide additional resources for co-operation. I envisage, for example, two to five full-time "ambassadors" in each jurisdiction, that can travel a lot in Europe, and that can make the connections across Europe about the results or the achievements that were made, or the mistakes that were made in each country.

We also need a couple of million Euros a year on translations. We notice that there is a lot of documentation around. But I am not able to read the documentations in Danish, in Swedish, or in Norwegian, or in other languages. So, if we have them translated into English, and if we are able to make a translation from English to each national language, then we have the first baseline; of course we need to process this documentation and assist the people in reading and selecting the documentation. But the very first step is to have a service for translation. It is really a trivial thing. It is feasible just with a small amount of money and we don't need a deep political involvement. Let us start with the trivial things, and then we go on with the more complex ones.

National Strategies in Centralized and Federal State Systems

Dr. Manfred Zipperer, Germany

We are concerned with national strategies in Germany. Mr. Paland and I have agreed that we will each present the strategic elements in Germany from the perspective of self-administration and from the perspective of the Federal Ministry of Health and Social Security Let me present the strategy of self-administration as follows : Health care in Germany is characterized by diverse decision-making levels and responsibilities. The medical care of the population is not in the responsibility of the central government or of the sixteen states, but primarily in the hands of the self-administration of health insurers and service providers commissioned by the government. They are active within the framework of statutory regulations, but financially and administratively independent. As a result, they have divided tasks which illuminate Germany's strategy from two sides. The government also establishes the statutory regulations within health Telematics. It appoints the leading organisations within health services to manage infrastructures and applications through agreements amongst themselves. The content of health telematic strategies is, therefore, strongly characterized by the ideas of the participating organisations. The Action Forum for Telematics in Health Care, which is organizing this congress, serves as a platform of consent for the self-administrating partners for the development of their own ideas and positioning in relation to political bodies.

Unfortunately, there are very few reliable examinations of the cost-benefit relations of telematic applications. The greatest savings are promised by the introduction of electronic prescriptions and the examination of the tolerance of medicines on the basis of a constant documentation of the medicines. The existing procedures are very costly and incomplete. The savings appear first of all for the health insurers as the investment costs are primarily carried by the service providers. A compensation for this must be foreseen in negotiations.

All experts have agreed that the application of health telematics will improve the quality of medical treatment. This applies not only to the documentation of medicines and the avoidance of double examinations, but also to an improved, immediately available and more comprehensive documentation of the course of treatment. Health data are highly sensitive data. Telematic applications will only be accepted by patients and service providers if they are secured and satisfy the particularly high standards of data protection in Germany.

The infrastructure and applications must be financed by the users, meaning by the health insurers and service providers, if possible with the participation of industry. Governmental support is possible, although not as a rule foreseen. Parliament has intentionally given broadly-drawn and technically-open framework conditions and allows the self-administering partners to shape them in co-ordination with industry, the sciences, patient representatives and data protection officials. The actors are foremost the associations of those carrying the costs and service providers which must implement the statutory regulations. They have to address industry and the sciences with their technical and organisational requirements in order to obtain their appropriate solutions.

The whole process of introducing a telematic infrastructure and its applications must be co-ordinated most closely with the federal and sixteen state supervisory authorities. This is also the deeper purpose of hosting this congress together with the Federal Ministry for Health and Social Security and the states, especially with the Free State of Saxony.

There are many model experiments and partial solutions in Germany. In my opinion, a national break-through is to be expected from two project commissions which the self-administering partners and the Federal Ministry for Health and Social Security have awarded. On the basis of their results, regional pilot projects will be launched starting in 2004 which should prepare the introduction and necessary infrastructure for electronic prescriptions by means of an electronic health card.

The motivation and readiness to improve the quality of treatment, to simplify the course of administration and in addition to this save money with telematic applications is high for all those involved. Opposition is to be expected because telematics increase the transparency of medical operations and because the allocation of resources is uneven. Financial incentives for the service providers will not be sufficient to make telematics a component of normal care. A comprehensive acceptance campaign is necessary to persuade all those involved that health telematics is of great use to them.

Norbert Paland, Germany

Networked information and communication paths are the necessary preconditions for cross-sectoral, integrated care and for more quality improvements, more efficiency, more transparency, and the strengthening of patient autonomy. This precondition will be achieved with the electronic health card. This will be the connecting link in German health care which connects over eighty million patients with approximately 270.000 doctors, 77.000 dentists, 2.000 hospitals, 22.000 pharmacies and over 300 health insurers. As such, it is the key to integration and co-operation reaching over individual institutions. The timeplan looks like the following: the introduction of the electronic health card is regulated in the Health Modernisation Law. This was passed on October 17, 2003 by the Second Chamber of the Federal Republic of Germany and can thus enter into force at the end of the year. This year, the conceptual groundwork for the card itself and the necessary telematic architecture and infrastructure will be prepared and performed. In 2004 the test phase will start which will lead to the implementation phase. In 2006 the electronic health card should be installed comprehensively. The Health Modernisation Law regulates the replacement of the existing insurance card through the electronic health card.

The new health card includes more technology and open, technical extensions to the insurance card. In order to enable the use of the electronic health card, rules will be made regarding procedures and standards and for the development and introduction of the information, communication and security infrastructure on the basis of a telematic framework architecture. The self-administration (*Selbstverwaltung*) should reach an agreement on a national level for the development and introduction of a comprehensive information, communication and security infrastructure which enabels and supports the use of electronic health cards. If this does not succeed, the legislature has foreseen a substitute solution ("*Ersatzvornahme*" by the Federal Ministry). The card must obligatorily contain the administrative data, the electronic prescription and the supplementary administrative data which correspond to the European rules for claims for services in the member states of the EU. Additionally, it should support, on a voluntary basis, the provision and use of medical data such as documentation of medicines, emergency data, patient receipts, electronic doctor letters, electronic patient files and eventually a data field for the insured which can be used by this person under his own responsibility.

In the area of patient rights and data protection, the consent of the patient and the right to read as well as detailed rules for access and a prohibition against use and seizure are to be determined. Through this, the greatest possible protection of the doctor-patient relationship is guaranteed and the acceptance of the health card considerably promoted.

Ákos Moró, Hungary

Today I learned a nice taxation system from Mr. Mori. If I try to put the Hungarian IT health care information system into this system, I think it is situated between the prototaxic area and the transition process. I will give you a very short review of the last years, of what has happened in Hungary and what founded our current strategy.

In the early 1990s, there were very serious structural and legal changes in the Hungarian health care system. This means that we changed the whole reimbursement system, we introduced the DIG based finance system in the hospitals, we introduced a German point system in the ambulant and outpatient system which includes a per capita reimbursement system in the GPs. There were the driving forces for information system development in the very early years of the nineties and which had been finalised at the end of the last decade. After this, in 2000, there was a new national scenario with a government programme which adopted the Hungarian information society strategy. In the context of the information society strategy, we created the health sector which is accepted by all relevant bodies and actors.

What is the current situation and what do we need to consider when we formed this strategy? There are a lot of sector strategies, needs from the social and economic environments, financial and business impacts, national and international trends. There are legal aspects, there are technological constraints, and last but not least there are the EU requirements. We need to see their internal SWOT analysis. SWOT is our strength and weakness. In the next steps, I would like to focus on the main objectives and the professional tasks and the current projects.

What are the aims of the strategy? The first is: individuals and communities must be properly informed about health and social needs related knowledge as well as information regarding the operations of health and social sector delivery organisations. That is the first objective or the first goal. The second one concerns responsible decision-making which must be based on appropriate, adequate and timely information. There are, of course, a lot of interdependencies in the different tasks – we are establishing the social info-communication conditions and infrastructure with an impact on health and social information knowledge, with both of them exploiting the health and social sector knowledge.

What are the main professional tasks? Very briefly: We would like to provide content services for health professionals and for the community, using Internet and telecommunication channels, with good quality public-professional health and medical information and knowledge. Secondly, we want to develop an interoperable health and social information system, with its infrastructure based on EU and international health IT standards. The third one is developing health and social indicators set reporting systems, a national health public database and the modernisation and the harmonisation of health monitoring according to European recommendations and international data providing WHO, OECD and some other agencies operate an Internet-based national health indicator database. And finally, encouraging and supporting the R & D sector and innovation culture is also our task.

I would like to show you the projects which we will try to develop in the next couple of years. The first – chronologically, not in priority – is establishing the health and the social sector web portal site. I must say frankly that there is a huge debate in Hungary regarding the difference between a web-site and a web-portal site. There is a functional difference between the two terms. The second one is establishing an Internet and call-centre-based public health information and patient system. Mainly, it is based on the UK type NHS Direct System, which was introduced, if I am not wrong, in Germany a few years ago. It was a very successful service. The third one is indicating the health indicator set, and we would like to strengthen the health monitoring system. The next project is that we would like to introduce eHealth term sets, eHealth IT standards and interoperable applications in Hungary. We will also try to develop the electronic certified public and social registries, e.g. for health and social services providing organisations, physicians, some medicaments or drugs and equipment etc. In the last decade, we also tried to implement a so-called hospital-based information system in a lot of Hungarian hospitals. Now we try to develop a regional public health information system which includes the hospital system, outpatient clinics, family physicians, the national public health system as well and the local authorities. We are also trying to establish and apply a digital signature in the health sector and in the social sector as well. There exists a timetable and a task-table which start in 2004 and will hopefully be finalised in 2006.

Dr. José Luis Monteagudo, Spain

I would like to present to you what is the current situation in Spain. We are forty million inhabitants and we have fifty million visitors. In all we have 17 regions which at this moment are all empowered to deliver health care. We are totally decentralized, and in this respect have health care such in a federal state. There are 800 hospitals and around 700 000 people working in the health system. The structure is in the hands of the 17 regions and the Ministry of Health with a top level of argreement by interterritorial councils. This co-ordinating framework is supported now by a very recent law on the "Cohesion and Quality of the National Health System".

What is special about the question of costs and benefits? The costs are often certain, but the benefits are very difficult to quantify in economical terms so most of them are estimated. Another point is ICT traditionally is established on a project basis. Decisisons are made project by project and not in reference to an overall framework. Most of the decisions are political, especially at this moment, with governments trying to stress the potentialities of modernisation in health care for their citizens.

The impact of eHealth is delayed in all the systems because it is extremely difficult to assess the real impact of investment, the real gains at the end of the chain. But talking about evaluation, we certainly need models, we need a new approach, we need to have information to support our decisions. We need to learn from the world. We try to understand what is happening, what is the information we can obtain from other experiences.

In our point of view at the moment, activities are only focussed on telemedicine. That is because telemedicine is a strongly connected with health care delivery. But what about applications for logistics or even for the electronic record? It is not appropriate to apply traditional health technology assessment to these elements. We have in fact results about telemedicine in all the projects since they are obliged to do a costs-benefits assessment. We have documentation about the

Canary Islands, about Andalucia and very soon about Galicia, too. And every year we have a call for such studies at our Institute.

All the regions agree that other qualities are connected with the law. The focus is on the patient-held results in proven assistance goals, the quality guarantee and the mobility for all the citizens. And what about participation, the empowerment of the patient? Obviously, data protection and confidentiality is one of the key elements. We are following European directives, but specific to the health care domain, we have national regulations for the health care records, patient autonomy and medical information. But a problem now is that seventeen regions have local regulations. So, you have a lot of conflicts, legal conflicts about how to perceive and how to harmonise nationally, not yet on a European scale, but internally. In this process, the most important elements are the e-commerce law and the regulation of the electronic signature. The electronic signature is now in the legislatory process.

What can be said about timescales? There are problems related to the medical elements. We can spend from one to three years because of the budgeting. If you are really fighting for a proper budget, it depends also on the political will. So if you look at what the amount of our expenditures in the system is, then we have to realise that implementation is on a theoretical basis. Typically, we record what the projects need and they are prolonged because performance is not as expected. What is really the time span for a project? Is it better to think about a continuous process including several projects or several budgets? We have to think and convince people that it is not a matter of projects, but a matter of developing a framework. Still, I will give you some real examples: the official schedule for developing a web-site for general public information in Andalucia is from February 2003 to February 2005. That means within two years there will be total change.

My next point is funding. I cannot refer to any real figure at this moment. We, in a general calculation, expect about one percent, in Galicia it is 0.9, and maybe this year in Castilla la Mancha it is 3%. But these are general figures, and they obviously are very low. The current budget of the ministry is for co-ordination and special projects. It is in fact very low, and I must say that the Ministry of Health is the last of the five. It provides the lowest resources in the general administration. But, in anyway we have this figure that our own is 15% this year.

Standardization is a traditional topic on the agenda of all governments. It is being intensively discussed at the moment and the search for solutions is going on. In a couple of years, we might have an organisation on the state level because interoperability is necessary to guarantee the mobility of citizens. And this is realised. Several regions have made some advancement: Galicia has submitted a regulation for DICOM and HL7 that is obligatory to pass before a committee. The Andalucian government is now establishing a similar organisation to regulate the standards for all the systems. Extremadura still is an open case because it adopted the open source platform LinEx for education, for government, and also for health care.

I would like to introduce some concrete project work to you. There is a lot of activity everywhere, but mainly in the infrastructural development of a network in the regions. All regions make their own local, regional, and national health records.

Telemedicine is flashy now. Every region is putting on telemedicine projects and health portals. There is another initiative in Andalucia for a high-level simulation programme for professional training.

What are the projects from the Ministry of Health? One is about the co-ordination, it is to support the health care information system. That, by law, is the responsibility of the central government. We are implementing a communication network that is started with all the regions. The Internet services for all citizenswere started recently, and also another portal for the centralisation of health alerts and an emergency network.

In addition, we are providing interactive services for health matters, and partly services for research management. Also we are working on telemedicine services for the future. In this line of preparation is a project which is preoccupied with the elderly and chronically ill patients. We have a network of research for this kind of telemedicine services and a special programme that I would like to explain a little bit more as an example. Its aim is to support chronically ill patients. The purpose is to create a path from research, from an original organisation to the national health service with three stages. The first one is with the primary project. Then we pass to a very brief evaluation in each region with a number of patients. That would comprise the methologies, clinical assessment, the cost-benefit-calculation under one modality that has been agreed between the regions. That is the controlled guidance of new technologies. And there is a budget for this kind of new technologies. And this line we also use for a special approach, that is co-operation within the industry. In this case, we have a contractor agreement with Vodafone and we are now entering with pharmaceutical industries into the other stages. The strategy is to diminish the risk of introduction into the market and to increase the number of population, of patients that enter in this forum.

It is important to provide trust to all the stakeholders that this innovation will be realised and a standardisation and a model of care will be agreed on. Agreement is not only needed about technology. Changing management is the issue. And, as we heard in the presentations today, we have the regions as leaders. eHealth definitely becomes a strategic issue, and all the top managers are aware of that. There is vivid activity concerning the problems of interoperability and harmonisation. Interoperability does not only refer to technical terms, it means agreement on the services, and on the general IT development in society. We only have 25% of the people with an Internet connection at home, 15% with broad band at home. We need 100% using Internet.

Mats Larson, Sweden

I will give a short presentation of the discussions we are running in Sweden. It is a very good initiative to present the various national strategies because it is important for us to learn from each other. And I surely will take some additional information back to Sweden from this conference. My name is Mats Larson, I am working with an organisation called 'Carelink', and I will just give you some brief information on what that is and also on the background of the current discussions in Sweden. I brought with me some information on the conditions in Swedish health care so that you can understand the framework that we are working with.

The Swedish health care structure is very decentralized. Sweden is a vast country, it has the size of France, but the population of Paris spread out in it. So there is a lot of space which is, of course, attractive; but it also creates some difficulties, e.g. when providing professional services such as health care. The organisational structure is based on 21 different county councils. They are totally independent, they make their own political decisions on where to go and how to finance the health care structures. They have the right to impose taxes on the population in the specific counties. And these organisations are not that big, they are not even close to e.g. the regions in Spain. A traditional or normal county council would have some four- or five hundred thousand inhabitants. So that is the size of these units that we are talking about. When you have a structure with independent actors, at least our Scandinavian or Swedish experience is, that these people immediately start to exercise this level of freedom and try to create a specific profile or try to develop a structure or a way of working that is slightly different from their neighbours. I think this is sort of a human experience. Of course, it also incites a lot of important development. But when it comes to ICT, it is not always and in all aspects positive. As we have patients moving around more freely for example, we need to have structures where these different organisations can communicate. And just to give you a brief view on some of the effects of this, I would like to hint at the amount of money, or the percentage of money, the county councils put into ICT. You can compare this to the figures you heard in the previous speeches. So there are some county councils that spend almost 5% of their total income on ICT, elsewhere there are others that use half of that level. And of course you will get very different structures, and very different ambitions in a country where these differences are so obvious. So, when this situation became apparent during the nineteennineties, there was an initiative to assess how we can at least increase collaboration and try to find some more common solutions when it comes to ICT in health care. That was when this organisation called Carelink that I am working with was founded. This was some three years ago.

I will briefly line out the discussion on ICT strategies that is actually going on in our country. But I thought it would be important for you to understand the structure and the decentralized nature of our health care system. Because when we started to talk about the pros and cons of having a national ICT strategy for health care, a lot of questions arose: Would this help, would this speed up the introduction of ICT in health care? We think we are fairly advanced, but of course we also have some areas where we need to move on much faster. Would such a strategy help to make the use of ICT meet challenges we have in health care, one of those being e.g. the lack of health care staff? In some parts of the country and in some specialities, but also more generally.

We meet a lot of patients' expectations to actually be able to provide information on a national level. Patients expect health care providers to have data available, regardless in which organisation the patients are seeking their services. These questions were discussed during the last year in our country. Contrary to some of the other European countries, the overall conclusion was that in our country it would be difficult to introduce a traditional model of an ICT strategy. And the main reason for this conclusion was the decentralized structure with these 21 county councils all on the same level with no superior organisation which could actually decide on a strategy, could make sure that it is implemented, could maintain the strategy, and most importantly, could support it financially. There were no voluntary actors or players that appeared during this discussion. I think one of the reasons might have been the fact that if you take on responsibility to introduce or form such a decision, it is also expected that you at least would have some idea or advice on how to finance the development. And that certainly didn't make that role more attractive.

So, what we decided recently was actually to try to develop these issues in a slightly different way based on some of our recent experiences. So we started to talk not about an ICT strategy, but about something that we have phrased an ICT infrastructure. Several of the previous speakers have used that term, and I think we have put a slightly different meaning to that word. Referring to an ICT infrastructure, we do not only mean the highways and the communication structure, but also security-models and methods for identification. There are also structures for information included in order to make an exchange of information beyond organisational boundaries possible. So that is a wider interpretation of the word infrastructure. When we communicate this with people in our own organisation, we use the picture of the highway system in Sweden. An ICT infrastructure would include the highways, but it would also include some of the services, some of the police services, some of the service stations, the gasoline stations, maybe even the motels. All that would be part of the infrastructure as well.

We think that it is important to start at one end, and what we have looked at now is how far have we come on this common ICT infrastructure. We, for example, identified the communication part where we have a national ICT health network in Sweden. We have a definition or specification for a common security model, using a PKI structure that is adopted to health care prerequisites. We have a model for identifying health care professionals. And we also have an emerging common information structure in place. So some of those basic elements that are necessary in an infrastructure are already there. But, of course, there are a lot of things missing. We think that in a later phase, in a couple of years, it will be important to add some of those more basic services as well.

One important aspect in our country is, and I am not sure what it is like in yours, that it is not likely to be successful if we try to centralize all these services. So what we actually try to do is to build on the decentralized responsibility, to use some of those specific skills. That would mean e.g. that the county council of Norrbotten, which is far north and very good at working with the electronic patient record, maybe it could take on the national responsibility to develop this service for the rest of the country. Norrbotten could hand responsibility for something else to another county council. This way you could actually distribute these national responsibilities to different actors all over the country. This is what we try to do with some basic services, and we think that this might in the future also be a model that can work in our system.

Just to give you one example, and this is important to know, just because it is one of the reasons why we in our country have decided to work in a slightly different way. Recently we concluded a project with the national Swedish health network, it is called "Sjunet". And this is an example of how the structure was built up in a very distinct bottom-up perspective. This project started in 1997 with only a small number of county councils coming together to form a regional network. But then in just a few years it grew because other parts of the country decided to join this system. This was a kind of development that we were not used to. It used to be that if someone did something interesting, someone else would do something slightly different. Just to distinguish. But in this case we got the positive development of actually having a joint structure. And in fairly short time this national structure was established. This was also to our satisfaction identified by the commission in the beginning of this year as one of the more interesting e-health initiatives in Europe Of course that made us very pleased.

I will give just a few examples regarding the use of this national structure and where it can make a big difference for patients. There is an example of a cancer treatment in one part of our country where you have the specialists in the University hospital and the patients and some of the staff living several hundred kilometres away. By using this national infrastructure, the service can be delivered without the patients' having to travel. Something else that is developing fairly rapidly now in Sweden is the use of video conferencing in health care. It is used very frequently as video consultations, involving patients, relatives and health care professionals. This also is a way to cover large distances, but it is also used just to improve communication. And we had experiences of using video conferencing in the old days, and in the eighties with the telephone lines. It is entirely different when you use an IT based network for this kind of services. That is our reason, that is our interpretation why it is catching on so rapidly now. Just a third example that raised some interest when we presented it in different places around Europe: We have a lack of specialists in radiology in our country and this causes a lot of problems, generates long waiting lines, and it also creates high costs to recruit staff. One of the hospitals in the northern part of the country, found out that there is an excess of radiologists in Spain – they are even unemployed. So by using this national broad-band network of Sjunet, and of course some other structures as well, they connected to a clinic down in Barcelona. And within three months' time they could reduce their waiting list by fifty percent. And patients started to come from other parts of the country to their little hospital in the north just because they had such an efficient way of dealing with the patients by using the specialists in faraway Spain. This is a very small example, but we found that it has been inspiring. A lot of other projects started which were modelled after this one. And this example is not any more a project, it has become part of their normal service, it is the way they deliver it to the public.

Here is another example, and I know that you in Germany are very engaged in electronic prescriptions. And that was a hot issue, an important issue, in our country a couple of years ago. But now it is our impression that we have this development in place. And we have five-folded the percentage of the prescriptions that are sent electronically, it is by almost twenty-five percent now. But still in some parts of the country the figure is almost 100%, once again due to the decentralized structure.

As a second phase, we have started looking at something that we have named a "common medication record". Patients have a tendency to go to different doctors and different doctors prescribe different drugs. Not always does the patient know or inform the doctor about the situation and of course, this creates a lot of problems, not only high costs for drugs, but also problems when patients use medication that is not prescribed with the knowledge of other, parallel, ongoing prescriptions.

So what we, with the use of this national information network, are working on right now is actually to have a "window" into each electronic patient record, where you can see all the prescriptions, regardless of whether they are made in primary health care, in specialised health care or even in another county council. So you get a complete picture of what the patient has been prescribed, regardless of where in the structure or where in the organisation. This is something that we think will save money on the drug bill, but also actually save the patients' lives.

Just to finalise, if you want some evaluation on cost-efficiency, of course, we are working on these issues just as all the other European countries do, and we found all the same difficulties in evaluating and in identifying the benefits. I just wanted to share with you an experience we had when we looked at how can you actually estimate the value when having a national health care network. How much money can you save? That is of course a valid question, but so difficult to answer. We took one of the twenty-one county councils and tried to study the effect there and tried to identify not only the obvious savings, but also the indirect savings, such as quality issues and a shorter waiting list. And this is the result that specific study. The investment of approximately 200 000 Euro on an annual basis is to support and to pay for the national infrastructure of that county council. If you consider only the direct benefits, you can see that the benefits exceed the costs. And if you add on the more intangible, soft values, it becomes even more attractive.

So this is one way of evaluating the benefits. These processes are important to use. At the same time, we find it very important to look at the benefits and the value from another perspective. And that is the patients' and the health care professionals' perspective. It is important to have them in mind all the time when we are working with these projects. The overall pursuit still is to work for a better health care. And we think that a national solution and national ICT structure can support that kind of development.

Marjan Suselj, Slovenia

I am going to outline the state approaches and the future strategy of the Health Care Infrastructure in Slovenia. I come from the Health Insurance Institute of Slovenia, which is the exclusive provider of compulsory health insurance at a national scale, so my presentation could be a little bit flavoured by the payer perspective. Over the past decade, we have been involved in the building of organisational schemes and different IT solutions in the country, and within this frame, we have achieved certain results; some of you are already aware of them, some of you will be today confronted with them. We are starting some new level of discussion on the entire health care system in Slovenia. Politics have decided to establish a health care reform, and I will address the topics of this reform which are important for the health information system.

In Slovenia, we have had a number of important achievements over the past few years. The electronic data exchange is the prevailing mode of reporting, and the intense computer support for the everyday work of health insurance and health care professionals has resulted in a high level of information technology literacy.

The health insurance card system was introduced to further integrate data flows in health care. The card system consists of a health insurance card, a microprocessor card distributed to every insured person and a health professional card serving as an access key to the network of service terminals and, of course, the IT platforms in the health care offices to operate the system. In the health care offices, the card serves as a source of current and up-to-date patient information. The computerised capture of patient data simplifies and splits up administrative procedures and the patient reception. The security scheme provides a major boost to privacy and security sensitive personal data.

The relevance of the system to the different user groups, in particular the citizens, is indicated by the progressively growing volume of transactions with the aid of the card system. The system not only supports the administrative and information tasks at virtually all health care offices, hospitals, health, medical and aid suppliers; in addition, the online terminal network also provides a number of services that traditionally required a visit to the nearest health insurance office. Upon its introduction in autumn 2000, the card system smoothly and quickly gained acceptance among all the user groups. In three years, the card has become common place. Today, the system has contributed to a high level of e-operation literacy among the Slovene population and health professionals. The purification of health data bases in the process of card introduction and automatic transfer of up-to-date, current data to the local data basis at the health care facilities has been a major step forward in the terms of data availability and accuracy.

Regarding the individual management of patients and their associated costs, a further important benefit is the reliable identification of patients and service providers in all contacts in processes in the health care system. In our national strategy, we pursue five main courses. The first one is the continual extension of information support to health insurance business operation. The second one is the progress in incorporation of medical data. In this field, a number of projects have been completed or are in process, and the examples are: recording of organ donorship commitment, information support for selected medical data to make them readily available in emergency situations, information support for the prescription and issuing of medical technical aids, and information support to medication. The next course is the strengthening of the autonomy of citizens in health matters. It is shown in the freedom to access their health related data whenever they wish to at an easy accessible service network. The number of services or enquiries supported by this network is progressively growing.

In view of the ongoing development of technology, the system requires continuous renewal and updating of technological components and the introduction of PKI is one of the main projects in the future. It is the last but not the least important segment of the integration of the Slovenian system into the EU infrastructure. Here, we are actively participating in some European projects.

So let us now address the most controversial issue in the public discussion in Slovenia: health care reform. The previous reform was carried out ten years ago. Slovenian politicians have assessed that the national health care system requires a far off review. The major impetus to advance to a new quality level is to cope with the present challenges in this environment. So the reform has been outlined in a Ministry of Health white paper. The white paper has awakened a vivid discussion in the professional and the general public. It set out six main objectives. I am going to address just two consequences of this reform which are important for ICT in health care. The reform of IT is also a segment of this reform as well. The efforts in this field are co-ordinated under a major project addressing health care systems management. This project is managed by the Ministry of Health and it is co-sponsored by the World Bank. The project objectives include the redefinition of the national data architecture, data models, coding systems and classification. Secondly, it includes the introduction of a case mix scheme in the accounting of hospital services and the further development of the electronic patient record and the setting up of a new national organisational and institutional structure to support health care infrastructure.

The new organisational structure is to be divided in three main layers. The first layer, the steering and governing layer, consists of a health informatics council at the Ministry of Health. It will consist of representatives of the high officials of all major actors: from the Ministry of Health, from the Health Insurance Institute, the Public Health Institute, and main health care organisations. It will co-operate with the corresponding council at the governmental level in the country. The council will be responsible to shape development orientations and to steer the work of the actors at the lower hierarchic levels.

The second layer will comprise ad hoc working groups mainly involved in the development of standards or technical guidelines. The third layer will consist of a project office. Its main task will be the co-ordination of know-how at the operational level and to combine the work of different outside contractors in the development.

At the end of my presentation, please allow me to point out some main findings that I believe will correspond to those in some other countries. The development of infrastructure in health care can only succeed as a continuous process -- not too slow, but also not too fast. There may be some outstanding individual steps, but these cannot be successful if they are not based on a previously existing infrastructure and a common philosophy. IT and infrastructure are merely tools for professional and business processes in the sector. They should adjust to the actual needs of the processes. Therefore, they are necessarily subject to permanent development and rebuilding. In the course of development, more and more actors and stakeholders will get involved. This makes the development even more complex and delicate in terms of establishing consensus and commitment among the ever-broader circle.

A last point: the international history of the development of IT solutions and infrastructure in health care exhibits a number of more or less successful attempts and efforts. It is obvious that, beyond national enthusiasm and activism, there is a definite need to share experiences and visions to avoid failures and to optimise effects.

Ivo Burger, Czech Republic

I come from the Municipal Hospital in Litomerice in the Czech Republic. It is quite near to the place we are holding our conference – only about 100 km south from Dresden. I am chief information officer in this institution, and this institution is known in the ICT field e.g. as the Macha project pilot site from the MACHA project and as the founder of MEDTEL.

My presentation will refer to three main themes. The first one concerns the perspectives of health informatics in the Czech Republic. Informatics in the Czech Republic is an integrated part of health care, it helps to carry out effectively all administrative tasks in the health sector. Secondly, I will hint at contemporary trends in information and telecommunication technologies, e. g. the expansion of nets, mobile technologies, improvements of hardware and software capabilities. – this is why information systems can be accessible anytime and anywhere with adequate security. Thirdly, the use of new information technologies in the health care sector depends on, maybe not only in the Czech Republic, but also in other countries, on finances, legislation and executives.

Another perspective is to focus on the benefits, on the assets the implementation of ICT brings about for the various participants. What are the assets of the new technologies in the health care sector? Assets of the new information technologies for health care providers are to facilitate patient data transmission and the provision of new tools and new diagnostic possibilities. This improves the quality of health care. Further assets for health care providers are the decrease of unnecessarily repeated medical examinations, the decrease of waiting-time for examinations, operations etc., and the improvement of diagnostics possibilities. This all brings us to price cuts and to the improvement of the quality of health care.

Another field where the new information technologies can be of advantage in the health sector is controlling. They enable a continuous evaluation of costs and benefits of health care providers referring to regions, hospitals departments, patients, diagnoses etc. The second application of controlling via IT technologies is the evaluation of the quality in health care. Statistic data from the region, hospitals or the whole state can be compared. The continuous control of financing and quality brings about more transparency in financing.

My next point leads to the transmission of health information. Prerequisite for all information systems is the protection of personal sensitive data.

In the intercommunication of the government information systems data sharing and data protection have to be ensured. There are two basic laws concerning the rights of citizens: they guarantee the citizen's access to all of his or her own records in government information systems and the possibility to initialize data updates. The safety key to data is the electronic identifier. It serves as verification for access to electronically safe data. It is a two key system. There is an electronic identifier of the health care providers and an electronic identifier of the health insured person.

One of our next tasks is to bring the electronic prescription on its way. It will be efficient in sharing registers, sharing safe interfaces and electronic identifiers.

Let me conclude at this point: the new information and telecommunication technologies and possibilities in health care allow to improve the quality of health care, they allow to compare the quality of the health care and its costs on a regional and on the state level, they add transparency to and thus improve financing. An important factor to be implemented now is the electronic identifier.

My next subject is MEDTEL MEDTEL is a large organisation in the Czech Republic. It means telematics in health care, following the definition of health telematics published by the WHO: “Health telematics is a complex term covering health related activities, services and remote data transfer systems operating via information and communication technologies, which are realised in order to support health, illness control, and health care from a general point of view, as well as to support education, management and research in health care.”

Why has it been established? In 1999 EHTEL was founded with the aim of organising a continuous democratic and neutral platform, where actors of different categories could meet and formulate together constructive approaches useful for all of them. The actors are considered authorities dealing with health care – the Ministry of Foreign Affairs, schools, research establishments – ; health care providers; health insurance companies; associations of patients, citizens and interest groups; business companies operating in the field of health care. MEDTEL would like to become a similar platform in the Czech Republic

What are the visions and strategies of this organisation? Based on MEDTEL’s experiences with the development, management and provision of telematics in Czech health care, and with regard to the trends in this field in the countries of the European Union, MEDTEL can become a basis of the national network of health telematics and, consequently, a partner for European organisations, particularly of the EHTEL network of health telematics.

I would like to outline the principles of the MEDTEL initiative: first of all it is the emphasis of the orientation of health care to patients, fully respecting their rights. It supports health organisations and employees in their aim to gain responsibility, to achieve economical results and to provide quality treatment. Futher it supports the provision of health telematics, which is an integral part and the prerequisite of quality professional activities as a tool for the development for those institutions. And MEDTEL promotes the rational integration at local, regional, national and European level, fully respecting cultural traditions and the independence of persons, as well as organisations.

MEDTEL is for everybody – organisations, institutions, companies and individuals – that is active in the fields related to health telematics. MEDTEL would like to be a platform, a forum, a club, which is open to everybody who is interested. Let me list a number of MEDTEL activities. MEDTEL regards as its taks:

- profiling itself as a permanent and continuous information source in the field;
- enabling meetings and discussions on the MEDTEL premises;
- organising telematics seminars, courses, trainings and workshops in the field;
- providing consultancy and advisory services in the field;
- regularly updating its site www.medtel.cz, so that this becomes a permanent source of up-to-date information. It is now available in English, too;
- maintaining active contact with the EHTEL association and others;
- annually organizing an international health informatics conference with a focus on the transfer of information about European and world activities in the field. The next one is on November 13th-14th;
- preparing suggestions, proposals and initiatives aiming at the development of health telematics in the Czech Republic, particularly within the context of European trends in the field.

The basic technical and organisational background consists of websites, established and operated by the Ministry of Health of the Czech Republic: www.medtel.cz, and premises at Lekarsky dum (Physicians' House) in Prague where negotiations and meetings can take place.

How can one characterise the concrete contributions of MEDTEL to development in health telematics? It serves as a permanent source of up-to-date information, it contributes towards the harmonisation of Czech health telematics with the European Union. MEDTEL offers the opportunity to exchange information, formulate requests and suggestions among all health care actors: be it a health care provider, a specialist in informatics, an institution, a patient, a state or regional administrative authority.

My last topic is a short presentation of the information system in our Municipal Hospital in Litomerice. Its implementation was started in 1993 covering the complexity of hospital, ambulances, radio diagnostics, biology, haematology, microbiology, economic and accounting departments and all other departments in the hospital. It then expanded in 1996 to up to 250 workstations; and it is a pilot site of the chip card project MACHA. Targets of the implementation of the hospital information system are the support of health care, the possibility of monitoring of health care, the monitoring of expenses and productivity, analyses and solutions, scheduling and solutions, support of research and education.

The project MACHA refers to smart cards in health care, health insurance and social welfare in the Czech Republic. Objectives of the pilot project were to optimise IT procedures, data structures, smart card facilities – security, European harmonisation and interoperability, acceptance of cards, cross-sector infrastructure.

Participants in the MACHA project were the ORGA Consulting GmbH from Germany, the Ministry of Health of the Czech Republic, General Health Insurance Office, the private companies APROKS Ltd. and IMA Ltd., international and local experts, the Municipal Hospital in Litomerice and six software houses.

The project was carried out in two phases, one from 1996 to 1997 was concerned with the basic functionality. Phase II from 1998 to 2000 aimed at the extension of the system to social security and pharmacy and tried to implement the electronic signature and security evaluation.

Phase I covered the preparative part, the data structure was determined, the setting base of patients / holders was located, the chip cards were personalised and distributed, the security of data was set up, a programme package was developed, the data terminal in the pilot site was implemented, initialised and verified. Phase II, the phase of extension involved the data of the national social security system into the data structure, the data structure on the chip cards was adjusted, the prescription was integrated into the data structure, the electronic signature was implemented, and the numbers of card holders and general practitioners were increased, the reception desk in the Municipal Hospital in Litomerice was built and introduced..

We now have 27 000 patient cards and 100 health professional cards and one personalisation equipment. Infrastructure consists of six health card reader stations in Municipal Hospital, nineteen health card readers at physicians', four health card readers at pharmacies, two stand alone card readers in ambulances and three information kiosks.

Let me just give a few hints about the data structure, the card provides 3k of memory capacity and contains 5 data blocks: the health insurant's identification data, the insurer's administrative data, the citizen's identification data for social insurance administration, the medical data of the patient, security data.

For the future we aim at a regularly evaluation of the current project, a step by step expansion of the infrastructure to cover the whole city, a review of the card's function at our pharmacy. The deeper solution of theme: the vaccination certificate, review of the medical data set, security and data protection and the multifunctional purposes of health cards.

The strategy for a nation-wide implementation mainly consists of three elements: the institutionalisation of Ministry of Health and General Health Insurance co-operation, the preparation of the board of co-operating institutions and the organisation of a series of promotion events.

Panel Discussion II
National Strategies in Centralized and Federal States

Mats Larson, Carelink, Sweden*; Dr. Manfred Zipperer,* Chairman of the Action Forum on Health Telematics, Germany*; Dr. José Luis Monteagudo,* Ministry of Health and Consumption, Spain*; Ákos Moró,* Ministry of Health, Social and Family Affairs, Hungary*; Dr. Gottfried Dietzel,* Federal Ministry of Health and Social Security, Germany*; Angelo Rossi Mori,*Institute for Biomedical Technology of the National Research Council, Italy*; Ivo Burger,* Municipal Hospital in Litomerice, Czech Republic*; Michèle Thonnet,* President of EHTEL

Moderator: Prof. Dr. Jean-Claude Healy, European Commission

Prof. Dr. Jean-Claude Healy

After having heard all the presentations, it is time now for questions to and answers from the speakers. Maybe I just start. I heard very often in the various presentations about the 'assessment' of IT implementation, especially in Sweden or in Slovenia. It is clear now, based on fact, but not based on a dream. Now we have demonstrated the substantial gains in productivity, access, and quality of care. Definitely this approach is absolutely mandatory for going ahead and convincing the decision makers. So, congratulations to Sweden, to Slovenia and to the others, for fulfilling the assessment of eHealth solutions. This was the bottleneck for the last four years, but now, based on facts, we can convince the decision makers how beneficial eHealth could be, and based on the Swedish data mostly, it is clear that the ratio might be: if the cost is one, the result is three. Something like that. Is that right?

Mats Larson

Yes, that is correct. I would like to bring up a slightly different issue, if I may. Maybe we should not only talk about our success stories, now that we have done that. Maybe we could just briefly touch upon some of the difficulties that I think none of us did highlight that in our presentations One of the lessons that we learned, or I have learned personally, is that the change process, as Angelo Rossi Mori pointed out, and some others commented on, is extremely difficult. It is possible to establish national structures when you are dealing with something that is new, that didn't exist from the beginning, because then it is often easier to introduce. It is an entirely different case when you have to make people change their solutions or their behaviour in order to implement a national structure. These are at least our experiences. In a decentralized structure like the one I described in Sweden, the autonomies of the different organisations are also reflected in the freedom of their different managers. And that is just as obvious in ICT as it is in other segments of health care. So, implementing a national structure in such a situation, to be very clear,, will definitely lower the degree of freedom of these regional managers ICT experts. And it will definitely create reactions. And this is one of the phenomena or lessons that we have learned during the recent years. As you move on with these new structures, and touch on areas where services are already in place, and you have someone giving up something in order to have a common solution, you will meet all stages of "resistance to change" regardless of what system you are changing.. It would be interesting to hear if this was specifically a Scandinavian or Swedish experience, or if it has to some extent appeared in other nations of this continent as well.

Dr. Manfred Zipperer

We have learned from the speakers, for example, that not only in Germany, but in Spain and in Sweden, that we have decentralized health structures. In Spain, e.g. there are autonomous regions, as far as health is concerned, and I would like to know: did these autonomous regions develop their own telematic strategy, or who has elaborated, if this was the case, a national strategy? Was it the government, was it a voluntary collaboration of the regions, or was it a third committee, or body, or whatsoever?

Dr. José Luis Monteagudo

In Spain, we have a general programme for the whole of the nation: Info XXI. It has been launched by the Ministry of Science and Technology and all the sectors are represented here. It is concerned with applications, mainly influencing the technological approach. But it covers only the health care aspect. Each region keeps the total competences about legislation, budget and programming of the information technology application in the health care domain. And so the concrete implementation depends on the region. In Andalucia, for more than ten years, there has been a strategic approach and they have established their vision step by step. Catalonia, which is a very developed region, has a very different structure. There are a lot of intermediate organisations, a lot of initiatives, a lot of very good projects, but there is not a written, stated policy.

All of the ten regions have proposed a special programme for health telematics. And all of them are proposing centralized patient health records. It is a national issue, it is on the table for discussion at this moment. We need some kind of agreement about the identification number. I really appeal to all the regions. So, there is a background of agreement, a table for consultation, an interterritorial body. That is the authority. That is a very challenging experience, and we try to overpass the difficulties of this kind of diversity. On the other hand, we have to positively note a lot of activity that is creative and gives us the opportunity to learn continually.

Marjan Suselj

The decision-making structure in Slovenia is a little bit more simple since the country is a very small one and we have just one insurance company. We have a certain number of experts and influential people. But even if the decision-making structure is very simple, decision-making is not necessarily simple. When we start some discussion in our project, we face many obstacles. I may just point one of it: health professionals' fear of being supervised. IT, of course, brings transparency, better control, and we spend quite a lot of time to establish a win-win relation with the health professionals so they now trust the system and trust those who are implementing the system. The same is true for the prescription segment of the health care process. We are spending a lot of time discussing the evolution of ePrescribing. Here the fear was also present and one excuse followed the other. In autumn 2003, a law established a new business role and the pharmacist is now authorised to change the generic original drug. Physicians require electronic prescriptions, because they want to have feedback information from the pharmacy. When we discussed this issue a year ago, they blocked the process of introducing electronic prescription procedure. So if we find the right time, the right incentive, then we can, of course, proceed.

Ákos Moró

Here is another similarity between Slovenia and Hungary: they are small countries with only one insurance. But there is no problem with the local authorities in Hungary; there are more problems with the professional chambers. They have their own, private initiatives and sometimes these are open initiatives; they are hidden initiatives. So we need to discuss with the medical chambers, and then find the right time and the right incentives.

Prof. Dr. Jean-Claude Healy

Maybe Sweden can respond now. What are the statistics in Sweden, answering the question mentioned by Germany?

Mats Larson

I would say that to some extent both the professional bodies and the patient and consumer groups have been driving forces in this development. I mentioned, even if I might have exaggerated it a bit, that some of these structural changes create reactions of resistance among ICT specialists;. Whereas the professional groups and the patient representatives, who can see the benefits from these changes, very often can be the driving forces, the ones motivating the investments. And we found this very useful. You have seen all these charts about whether it is one, two or three percent that we, from the overall spending on health care, use for ICT investments. And of course, this is never enough. But by involving the professional organisations and the professional groups, it is more realistic to have the discussion about the 97% of the spending that is used for all the other costs in health care. This makes ICT a respected or a recognised cost just as the expenditures for drugs or other necessary items in our sector. And we have seen some very positive aspects of this change that surprised us a lot. Where health care professionals would come out and say: "we need to invest more for data protection and ICT security, and we are actually able to provide the funds for it".

Dr. Gottfried Dietzel

When the programme committee designed this international day, we focused on strategies, and we wanted to learn whether there is a difference in strategies in federal systems or in centralized systems. How do you design a strategy? You can lean it upon the technological development, the organisational development and the quality. And you can try to combine different forces within and by a strategy.

If I look at the results in the different countries, I notice there is really no difference between federal systems and centralized systems. And independently of this, we have similar key issues: ePrescribing, the use of cards, electronic health records, the building of regional networks. These are combined activities.What really is of interest, if a country starts these activities, is: What are the barriers? What about acceptance?

It would be nice – maybe this is work either for an EHTEL working group or for a follow-up conference – to concentrate on questions of acceptance in regard to certain applications. I am curious to learn why a certain card development worked in one country and did not in another. You are very successful in Slovenia and I would like to discuss that more in detail with you; on the other hand, as I understood, the Czech effort with the Macha card was not continued. It was a similar set-up of the card, but why was this development stopped and not continued? What are the different experiences? If I see now this picture in an individual country and the European development, then I must notice that when we designed the European card, we didn't actually take into account all these experiences and the knowledge that we could have gained from our national experiences. So maybe when we design the next step of the European card, we should go back to the national strategies and see what we have learned from the national projects. So coming back to our overall questions – what can we learn from national experiences – there is really something to learn that we can integrate into a European development in this field.

Prof. Dr. Jean-Claude Healy

Let me make a short comment before transferring the floor to Mr. Rossi Mori. It is clear that, ten years ago, the problems were technology and added value. Five or six years ago, there was a problem of cost, what is a matter of investment, ongoing cost and so on. Afterwards, it was a problem of methodology for assessment. The problem today and tomorrow is user acceptance. So, the implementations are guided by these three different steps: technology, cost or investment, assessment and human acceptance. Some countries are in advance, others are not. Nevertheless, all the countries have to follow these various steps of implementation.

Angelo Rossi Mori

I would like to bring my experience or my impression from Italy. In my view, the major factor that guided our decisions in Italy is fashion. It is not reasoning, we don't have a debate and thus we don't have the criteria yet to decide. We have the booking centres. This is a keyword. Everybody is implementing booking centres at the level of the hospital, at the level of the municipality, and now at the regional level. Because it is something that people can understand.We start to form the solutions that are understandable, not the solutions that are cost effective or something like that. So, there is no cost-benefit study behind these solutions.

What the people are able to understand is a solution that is practical, that is visible. So we have the fashion of the booking centres. From the eGovernment effort, we took the electronic signature which is being introduced in health care, we took the networks. Everybody is making networks everywhere in Italy now because it is the fashion. Everybody is speaking about broad band, but not about the content that will travel through the network; we have a number of decisions that are induced by things that are not really scientific or related to rational criteria.

About the cards: we wondered about having the laser cards, we had the chip cards, we recently had the bar code on the card– without any electronic mechanism. We don't know how to make the decision. Now we want the identity card. Then we want the health card, either with a content or only for identification. There is no real criterion, because there is no real debate. And, for eGovernment, I never heard about a cost-benefit analysis. The decisions of the national and regional governments, in Italy at least, I don't know about the other countries, are never, never made on the basis of a cost-benefit calculation. We know what to do. It is obvious. It is common sense. We need a better bureaucracy, we need to simplify all the paperwork etc. There is an obvious benefit. I cannot understand why in our case we have to demonstrate that there is a benefit. Everybody understands that reducing bureaucracy makes everybody's life easier, regardless of the topic. But in health care, people do not understand what the benefit of an electronic health record is.

Most people don't know how to deploy the electronic health record across the country. So, in my view, it is a problem of explanation, a problem of stimulating the fashion and increasing the awareness. It is not an economic problem because, when people understand, the money arrives.

Statement from the audience

Thank you for this very informative presentation. I have two questions: one relating to Mats Larson's regional problems which we certainly share in my country, which is Denmark, you know that well. And with us I think it is not the IT people so much as the professional people who shift the role when we introduce eHealth. Because it is not only a matter of transgressing the local border, it is a matter of going global and some people are scared of that. But in this context, although we had all these bright presentations, I am missing really the impression of the UK, or England rather. think we should not forget that this is a country that massively invests now, apparently with a strategy, putting 2.3 billion extra pounds into the health care system in three years. It is a massive effort. And I would like to compare Mats Larson's regional approach with the UK approach. In my view, the strategy is formed in order to get money, simply in order to finance the system. Mats has, and at home I have systems where the regions pay and decide. And the UK has one huge national employer, in contrast to anybody else. And I would like to know what do they expect, what are their experiences, would there be anybody in the audience who would be willing to give a comment on that because I think that would be interesting.

Statement from the audience

The UK situation, I think, is very different in the one respect you talked about. Somebody said eGovernment doesn't have business cases in the same way. This is certainly true in the UK. They are only now building the business case for the national programme. You will have seen maybe the McKinsey report recently which said that if they had done it on a regional basis, and everybody had done their own thing, it would have cost them ten billion pounds more than the money they put in. Now, if you believe that then there are pigs flying outside. OK. Nevertheless, the principle is that most of the national programme is predicated on political imperative. They have to do this or the health system in the UK will fall apart unless they have an electronic infrastructure to support it. You cannot have the source of systems that we require for citizens without a life-long electronic health record. The difference is that somebody has said, and we think it is Tony Blair, they are going to do this because, if they don't, the consequences are too awful for him to get re-elected. Now, they will build the business cases back from the other end. But I think that is the difference and that perhaps is an opportunity for all the other countries who are more fortunate or less fortunate, depending which way you look at it, in structure. Looking at the processes and how they get on with it, it will not be straightforward. We have identified some problems like: the big companies which are bringing in the provision of these services, but do not have an adapt knowledge of the health domain. The small companies have the knowledge, but how do they fit in with the big ones? This is a very strong current problem which you will all face, because you need all of the companies – little ones, new ones, big ones to make this happen. And the way of bringing all of these results together, getting everybody to work together in the same direction, is one of the key issues. Does that answer you question?

Prof. Dr. Jean-Claude Healy

Thank you so much, very clearly and demonstratively. Maybe you, Mr. Burger, can comment on the previous question about the MACHA project, please.

Ivo Burger

The project MACHA was closed for a general insurance company, but not for the Municipal Hospital in Litomerice. It was designed only for small partitions, not for a country level at the start position, it could expand to the whole country after that, after pilot examination in this project. Now there are proposals from some industry companies to general insurance companies regarding how to arrange the implementation of the smart card or another card in the Czech Republic. The main problem of all is the money at the beginning of the implementation. Everybody knows that these cards bring to us benefits, but there is not enough money at the start. It also depends on legislation; we have not prepared any good laws for it so far.

Statement from the audience

I wanted to add that IT companies are trying to make some applications with the card, raising the knowledge and the information.

Ivo Burger

In the Czech Republic, there is now no problem with hardware and software and public or professional acceptance – the problem is the financing at each of the levels as I pointed out.

Prof. Dr. Jean-Claude Healy

Finland, welcome the former President of the health telematics group.

Hannu Hämäläinen

I have two questions. First, I couldn't find the role of the private companies, especially the ICT companies, in developing RNB. Actually, I think that business strategies are tackling most of the difficulties of implementing IT in the health domain. And perhaps that was the reason, but anyway I think there could also be some reasons and problems to discuss. I think that in many countries, in ours at least, the IT companies have rights and, of course, business interests in this area. Not just in the implementation of health products in the health domain, but also in developing new services and facilities for us. How do you see that it is just the implementation and not the co-operation in RNB in this field in your countries and strategies? The second question comes from that they sound very nice, the problems and success stories, the cases where the ownerships are clear. I mean with the ownership that we are implementing IT in the health domain, and especially the cases that, also in other branches, are available. Eighty percent of the IT implementations today happen in re-organising the processes inside the organisations. The same applies to the health domain. How do you see the new consumers, the new citizenship, the new ownership of health? Very often in new e-commerce, we find user-oriented services where the citizens and patients are not just normal users. And that is a weak strategy point in our national policies, because the ownership is missing. We can see some other cases where we have central systems – it is hard to see.

Prof. Dr. Jean-Claude Healy

Thanks. Who wants to comment? Who wants to respond? Sweden?

Mats Larson

Yes, I would like to comment on the last question. The fist one I didn't really get. When it comes to consumer interest and influence, what we see in a growing extent is that both young and old patients or citizens are being driving forces for structural changes. And I think that is similar in many other countries. Patients expect to be able to have their medical data available, wherever they are in the country, for example, and they are highly surprised when they realise that the information that was fed into the system in one hospital is not available in another hospital. Because that is the way they expect the ICT systems to work. However, since this is not the way it works in our domain think that this expectation is a very powerful and useful tool to support change. To introduce some of the new services and some of the necessary alignments, you have to make this transition of national or cross-country information-flow work.

Prof. Dr. Jean-Claude Healy

Thanks. Who wants to comment on the first question?

Statement from the audience

I would like to add this reflection: yes, the end-users, the consumers, are those who require new services. However, the infrastructure itself is usually taken another way. One insured person doesn't know which network, which technology has to be established, but those entities that were responsible for the organisational insurance schemes, or health provider schemes, do. Those entities have to take some measures and it's their responsibility to establish the basic infrastructure. When the infrastructure is in place, then there is no question where we would want to go, because users require new services. But the basic infrastructure, from my point of view, is the task of those entities which are responsible within the countries to establish health care. Maybe I come back to the question that has been raised before: what were the success factors in our country? Definitely the commitment of those people who are responsible and felt responsible to establish the infrastructure, with the money, with the decisions and with a lot of courage, of course.

Statement from the audience

I would like to prolong your statement. To set up IT in health care in a country, there has to be someone who is really interested in IT and who really sees the benefit of it. The reason why it is understood is another issue, probably there is not enough money in the system, or probably, like in England, someone would like to be re-elected. But I think there really has to be someone who really understands, who pushes these ideas, and who has the power to get it to the right action. What I am missing in this discussion is the French example. Are there any IT issues in France?

Prof. Dr. Jean-Claude Healy

Ms. Thonnet, acting not as chairwoman of EHTEL, but as a member of the French Ministry of Health.

Michèle Thonnet

Thank you for the question. I will switch to my position in the french health ministry. On this issue, I agree with the Slovenian point of view that we have to have a national infrastructure first. And in France, as some of you may know, we already have this kind of infrastructure. We decided five years ago that the first and most important point is to build up the infrastructure. We did this in the way I have explicated. We don't think that it is enough to have this infrastructure, we have also built some new services on security, like identification, authentication, digital signature etc. In 1993 we set up two specialised national agencies, one (the GIE SESAM-Vitale) dealing with the Carte Vitale, the insurance card for every citizen in France, and now not only for every French person, but for every resident in France. The second structure (the GIP CPS) was created for the CPS card, the card for the health care professionals. It is introduced now; I can report that, some years ago, we had plenty of articles in the newspapers, but nowadays, nobody speaks about it. It is simply done and in daily use.

So we are on the second level. We have build and deploy this infrastructure, we begin to have an info-structure, dealing with semantics, coding and applications (administrative and medical ones). From January 2004 on, we are supposed to have a new coding for medical acts, It will be a common one because at the moment we have two, one for GPs, and one for hospitals. Another aspect is how to deal with e-prescription. It is not so obvious like we heard about Slovenia or other countries because France is a little bit different in the European Union. This is to say, we like to have freedom, a large degree of freedom. In France, we don't have any gatekeeper, you can go to any doctor, to as many doctors as you want in fact, and you will be reimbursed for these visits. Concerning pharmacies, you can go around the corner to have your prescription filled, but you can also choose to have this drug at another corner. We are not ready at the moment to build a repository and be able to set up this e-prescription and new procedure because it is not covered by the law. But, because it is so difficult, we decide to move a little bit away from this, from health care professionals, especially medical doctors and pharmacists only closer to the patient.

We are now building on the new "patients"law which was voted in March 2002 expressing the right for the patient to be more responsible and the owner of his medical record whether it is a paper one or an electronic one. We are now writing a decree on behalf of this law saying that each person could go even outside the hospital, even outside the medical doctor's office, and have his medical health care record in electronic form on behalf of a special structure that had to be accredited before. It was a really big issue because we have launched two years ago a consultation, regarding the possible recommendations to implement the "patients" law, in order to take into account the position of all the stakeholders.. Since some months, we have real pressure from them and especially from patients and citizens. Now we are beginning to have an interesting consultation with the interested industrials partners in order to set up this new system for the full benefit of the patients.

Prof. Dr. Jean-Claude Healy

Thank you, Ms. Thonnet. The situation is changing, but in a positive sense. How many cards are distributed in France, how many millions? 46 million Euros, so this is substantial. OK, Switzerland.

Statement from the audience

Reflecting these presentations and these costs, we are swinging between polarities: centralistic aspects, decentralized, and also acceptance or resistance. So my question is: where is the winning formula? Mats Larson pointed to one, but we have failures, too, and not only success stories. This is not only combined with expected resistance, with people; in fact, they are concerned stakeholders, people have their fears. We can, of course, impose any strategy, but it is a matter of efficiency to be successful in a more smooth way. So, how to seduce people, how to win those people? After that, there are the questions of how to create trust and credibility. So I would be interested to hear something about your personal experience on how to win people, on how to be more efficient in creating trust and credibility, and then be successful with those projects?

Prof. Dr. Jean-Claude Healy

This is really relevant with that newly updated question of user acceptance. Who wants to respond? Maybe Sweden?

Mats Larson

I think that that is a very important issue that you bring up. As I already commented, my personal reflection would be to stimulate a much larger degree of involvement from the medical professionals. We have a tendency in the ICT-domain to "develop solutions, and then go and look for the problems". I think that is one of the reasons why we have a history of some failures and some difficulties.

One way to move forward is to change the perspective and, to a larger extent, build on the needs and the demands of the medical professions – e.g. nurses, doctors, physiotherapists. To move forward in a more clear way we need to use their needs and expectations as driving forces rather than the ideas, challenges and priorities of the ICT people.

Statement from the audience

The question you raised is one of the essential questions when introducing ICT technologies, especially when you have in front of you the entire population, with different educational levels, with different expectations. I think there are no other ways than to work with them, to work systematically. It takes time, of course, when we provide a certain novelty. We combine different approaches, with information published through different channels.

With the focus on Europe, we provide media information at the local and the national levels. Of course, it is very important to establish a kind of call centre with supports which promptly answers all the problems which could occur. And, of course, all this needs resources.

Prof. Dr. Jean-Claude Healy

A bunch of systems and services are planned to be implemented within the next few years. And I am sure, within the next three or five years, the third generation of mobile product technology will be integrated more intelligently and more quickly. So it is symptomatic of the dynamic eHealth approach, and thanks to

Euroview, to the so-called AIMS community Niels Rossing established 12 years ago, this community is vivid now, and acts as a community. I am sure that the future will be based on eHealth solutions. Thanks to all of you.

Prof. Dr. Jean-Claude Healy

National Strategies as Structural Elements for a European Telematics Strategy

The objective of this presentation is not to educate or to inform: you are very well educated, you are very well informed and aware of everything. But maybe I can present a tentative, synthetic approach about the past, about the present, and about the future. With your agreement, I will focus on a development for all of you, based on research and non-research, and maybe I will focus on the non-research component support to implementation.

Here we are. We are just in the middle, we are in the centre. During the last fifteen years, the Commission has supported research activities in the domain of information society for health care purposes and allocated roughly 500 million Euros from 1989 up to the year 2002. This is a lot. What the global output of this very large initiative is we can say in short, definitively is sure now. A third industrial pillar exists, the eHealth industry, and this industry is very dynamic in Europe and very promising for the future.

We in Europe, for the moment and for the future, for the next ten years, have to completely revise our strategy. Not just to continue during the successive framework programmes, to support the same approach in health care. The first concept is to move from information technology towards knowledge technology, and from the health care approach to the health approach. For doing so, we have to split our activities into two components. The first component is research, and the second component is support to implementation. First of all, the research component. Quickly, during the Sixth Framework Programme, we developed integrated programmes based on user needs. We located a lot of products, in particular in the HINE proposal managed by Deloitte and Touche.

What about the market for eHealth? Other proposals were funded, including PRO EHTEL, for merging together the shareholders of the games and others. TM-Alliance for example, merged together the European Space Agency, the International Telecommunications Union, and welfare organisations. IHE-E, for example, managed by the European Co-ordination Committee of the Radiological and Electromedical Industries (COCIR) merged together large industrialists and they put in place the famous 'connectatron' demonstration, showing that all the products could be physically interoperable and so on and so forth. Finally, the Fifth Framework Programme is near to completion at the end of 2003. We thus await the final assessment of the programme.

In the Fourth Framework Programme, we developed the so-called flower model, relating societal demands. The demands of the citizens changed recently; in the past, it was essentially hospitals, patients and so on. But definitely now we have to focus on the domain of the citizen. The demand of the patient is to be cared for in the best possible way and the demand of the health professional is to optimise the human, technical or financial resources with regard to the health system. For each one of those three petals of the flower, a lot of information technology could be relevant as a matter of health supplies, web services, telemedicine services, home care monitoring, etc. This flower model was used as a basis for the Fourth Framework Programme.

But, what is maybe really essential is that one of the outputs of the Fifth Framework Programme is the so-called access, quality, economy (AQE) model that can be used for assessment. Ten years ago, we tried to apply in the eHealth area the classical methodology for assessment of biomedical informatics. It was not so successful, because we are concerned by diffuse technology. And we have to boost, to check properly, both the local impact and the structural impact. If, for instance, a product is cost beneficial for the social security system, the doctor doesn't want to implement it. Or, the reverse, if a product is very useful for the improvement of the quality of care, maybe it will be more expensive and the social security system will not accept to pay for it.

So, finally, after a lot of discussion, we decided to encourage the so-called AQE model in "access to care" in an effort to convince the politicians, who are very sensitive to citizens and about "quality of care", in an effort to convince the users and the doctors, and in "economy of care" in order to convince the financial authorities. So this model uses three components. These three individual variables must be checked out in a completely different way in the various member states or local authorities. Of course, each of them must be checked, but we cannot impose a single granularity of scale.

What means access to care in Sweden? What means access to care in Germany? What means access to care in Slovenia? I don't know. You know. So based on these independent variables, you can adapt yourself the granularity and the scale of the methodology of implementation. This is absolutely essential for the preparation of the future. All member states and regions must have a methodology for assessment, but we should adapt this concept to the local system.

The global output of research into eHealth was clearly manifested during the award process presented during the last eHealth ministerial conference in May 2003. In particular, there was an award for a network, an award for health professionals, and there were some awards for the patients and for the citizens. Sweden got one of them. Congratulations.

Now, in the context of the new Sixth Framework Programme, we are changing our prime orientation to knowledge. The first question is: where is the knowledge in biology and in medicine? Globally, knowledge is diverted in three different scales: the macroscopic scale, based on electronical informatics and concerning electronic health records, medical imaging etc. The scale is a metre. The second level is the opposite: the nanoscale, molecular scale with genomics and proteomics. A lot of knowledge exists in this area, but, for the moment, it is a matter of extraction of knowledge. In the middle, on the cellular or the tissue level, on a microscopic scale, a lot of knowledge exists – for example, this is true in nEuro-informatics – what is my way of thinking, my way of warning, my way of organisation etc.

So the overall objective of the next ten years' activities, and not just the Sixth Framework Programme, in eHealth will be to facilitate interoperability between these various, heterogeneous and disseminated databanks. The work will be to develop interfaces and the best possible components of common functionality between macroscopic, nanoscopic and cellular scales. This is what is extremely challenging, merging together a lot of different sciences, biological science, nEuroinformatics science, medical science, semantic science, thermodynamic science, mathematics, and including philosophy, semantics, and medicine. Be aware of this very, very enormous challenge. I am sure that, as a part of the Seventh Framework Programme, something will be developed in this area. For the short term, we have to facilitate the merging of the various data banks – heterogeneous, non-structured, distributed, with strong data protection – with one and another.

In addition, always in this domain of research, we can transfer the very efficient "Six Sigma Approach", previously developed by the company, General Electric (GE). During the last two centuries, we focused on the health care system. The magical words were hospital, patient, treatment, drugs, and doctor. But we can demonstrate that if we invest one penny or one Euro, the return is not guaranteed due to the complexity. On the reverse, we can duplicate the efficiency of manufactured protocols developed by GE by expanding the Gaussian curve up to six sigma. In the one direction, it comprises the basic components of genomic and personal data and personal risk factors. The second level is personal risk management – what about my diet, my behaviour, etc. And, globally, we go to early detection, professional risk management, home care monitoring, continuity of care, public health risk management and policy.

By expanding the scope of the health initiative, maybe we can substantially improve the overall efficiency of the elevated health system in comparison to the traditional health care delivery system. And as a trend, this one is very sensitive because it focuses on the individualisation of treatment and is based on citizen responsibility, activeness and pro-activeness. Maybe this is for the mid to long-term perspective as it is a substantial change in the re-engineering of the system. Immediately, we have to integrate this updated situation by conceiving new technology, intelligent technology, in order to facilitate for the patient, for the citizen, and for the family, personal risk management, community risk management, etc. So the Six Sigma Approach is, just as in the beginning, a plan to move from health care to health, from patient to citizen and it holds a lot of enormous consequences as a matter of infrastructure.

Globally, once again, we launched the first call for research submissions in the Sixth Framework Programme in November 2002. In May 2003, we selected twenty-one proposals out of 175, demonstrating the popularity of the domain. The overall request for our projects was 1.2 billion Euros, of which we can just pay roughly 90 million Euros. But this fact is symptomatic, not just because of the maturity of the domain, but also because of the popularity the eHealth domain has gained by now. We are absolutely impressed by the number of proposals that we have received. For the moment, in December 2003, we are undertaking negotiations of proposals.

What is new is that we have revised a little bit our methodology for implementation of research. During the Second, Third, Fourth and the Fifth Framework Programmes, we based our investment in projects where 50 % was paid by the consortium and 50 % was paid by the Commission. The efficiency of this methodology was not perfect., We now try to change our investment through the use of so-called integrated projects and networks of excellence.

An integrated project that we will be supporting is, for example, research on intelligent clothes. The commission paid sixteen million Euros, which is a lot of money, with a large consortium managed by industrialists, with a definite guarantee of results. So, an integrated project is an industrial approach with as much as possible a guarantee of results.

On the other hand, the so-called network of excellence, is a guarantee of skills which merges all the excellence centres in Europe or worldwide in order to accelerate knowledge in the domain of nEuroinformatics or some other such field.

So, two different instruments, Integrated Projects with the guarantee of results which is an industrial approach, and Networks of Excellence with the guarantee of skills with much more of an academic and traditional research approach. We continue to use the specific targeted research projects (the new name for the more traditional research and development projects), but gradually the proportion of the share of financing allotted to these types of projects will move from 20% now to zero.

So, definitely as a trend for the future, Integrated Projects and synergy will be the instruments. In line with this research, we are impressed by some inefficiencyies during the previous funding. For example, during any framework programme, we allocated ten, thirty, forty million Euros for providing, for example, classical medical help for cancer institutes. The return is extremely poor in general. Why? Because we pay for a big, big computer from a very clever and excellent centre somewhere. A few years later, the centre has no more money after the contract has finished. They have no more money for upgrading the computer and no money for paying for software and so on. The return is not good. We decided to stop any dedicated funding in this domain.

We are using the European infostructure named Géant to merge together all the member states from 2.5 up to ten Gigabit per second. So, already, the Géant infrastructure exists between all these member states based on this technical infrastructure. We develop great infostructure based on common middleware, for example, metabrowsers, many sophisticated forms of middleware common to nuclear physics, meteorology, freight mechanics etc. They are common and they are regularly updated in a purposeful way.

At the top, we can add a thin layer of HealthGrid dealing with data protection and confidentiality,. So we expect, within the next five years, that every excellenc centre, any research hospital, any cancer institute can plug in and use a high speed computer, whatever it is, with a very, very updated middleware, in open source. Investment costs will be peanuts and the running costs will be peanuts. So we are now revising our strategy and we strongly propose the so-called

HealthGrid. Already we have two or three projects that are supported by the Commission in order to test the feasibility of this concept. And please, please, each of you, associate with and promote the HealthGrid. Maybe the health area will be the first to be implemented by the Grid. It is very essential for political reasons, for technical reasons, and for efficiency reasons.

Other topics for research could be, for example, intelligent clothes, which I mentioned before, in referring to a large integrated project co-ordinated by Philips that will merge all of this new intelligent clothing industry.

The third, very interesting topic is biomedical informatics, which is related to the extraction of knowledge on nano, micro- and macroscopic scales.

Concerning eHealth itself, we plan to launch a call not before December 2004 and the deadline for evaluation will be around February 2005. We again plan to allocate roughly 100 million Euros' co-funding. But, in addition to the classical eHealth call such as this one, many, many Sixth Framework Programme calls are launched every three or four months in macro- and nanotechnology, and embedded systems. Many calls concern directly or indirectly eHealth.

More important now is the support given to implementation. Last May 2003, the first eHealth Ministerial Conference was organised in Brussels with the help of the SANCO Directorate-General. The output of the conference is clear, it is a Ministerial Declaration. All the ministers present invited the member states to implement and the Commission to facilitate the implementation of eHealth. Based on the output of the Ministerial Declaration, we got the mandate to go ahead.

Three or four years ago, we developed an analysis of where we are in the domain of integration of IT in the system. We developed a Sigma curve, a learning curve, with three components: one is IT specified gadgets, two is a Trojan horse, and three is to merge all IT components together. Finally, as a part of part three, the process itself is completely re-engineered as a matter of process, hierarchies, salary, recruitment, responsibility etc. For example, around the nineteen eighties, in manufacturing as it was before IT, we needed maybe two or three days to make a car. But with the full integration of IT in manufacturing, we now need just half a day. This learning curve was applied to the manufacturers system in IT in the nineteen nineties in business activities; now, it is applied in non-profit areas such as health, education, governments, and so on.

When we benchmarked IT developments in the year 2000, it was a hypothetical assumption on the impacts of IT. It is however no longer IT for quasi-doctors; everybody is now concerned – patients, citizens, health care authorities, finance directors etc. The key point is: it is not the duty to develop IT technology to aid the existing health care systems, but to anticipate phase number three which is the re-engineering of the system based on the citizen, based on free movement, knowledge and so on. This learning curve is a very good instrument for drafting the future.

This is why we invented the so-called European eHealth Area. There was a reminder during this conference that there is no mandate for health care at a European level. So the SANCO Directorate-General has no mandate in the domain of public health, no mandate in the domain of implementation. On the contrary, the Commission has a mandate for research, for support of the economy, for employment, and - via information technology - particularly for eHealth. It is why we designed the concept of a European eHealth area; it is eligible. I highlight what the instruments available to facilitate implementation are: one is an administrative instrument. On May 5th in 2004, during the Second eHealth Conference, organised by the Irish presidency in Cork, the Commission will announce a Communication. Communications are one of the instruments which make member states aware that a policy or a development exists. We shall invite you to act in this way.

The next tools are legal instruments, for example, the mobility of patients. We have to be cautious and not use this mobility too much; but de facto, the mobility of patients is a powerful instrument for merging together a lot of data.

The technical instrument in particular is standardisation. Standardisation is the responsibility of the Directorate-General (DG) on Enterprise. In addition to the eHealth conference in Cork, there will be a satellite meeting on May 7th 2004, organised by DG Enterprise not for standardisation, not for facilitating the way of standards implemented by TC25 etc., but based on a guarantee of result interoperability. The new trend for DG Enterprise is to guarantee results and interoperability within a short period of time. The satellite meeting with the participation of industrialists will be organised by DG Enterprise.

We try to collect together all the financial instruments available. We cannot predict how much money exists. In the research field, you can say - for four years - 200 million Euros. It is good, but it is peanuts. For the structure, we have roughly 40 billion Euros a year. The support of eHealth infrastructure is eligible to be funded through the structural funds. Unfortunately and stupidly, due to the lack of demand, part of these funds are not even used. That is why maybe, during the eHealth conference, a document will be distributed regarding which type of funds could be used: structural funds, indirect funds, or metafunds in order to facilitate investment as a matter of infrastructure, as a matter of services or additional initiatives. In addition, we have now the DG SANCO Public Health funds, but once again 300 million Euros divided over five years. It is peanuts. The money from DG SANCO is very rare. The money provided by DG REGIO is very easy to get and not so rare.

Finally, the last tools to highlight are educational tools. This line is urgent now and not only as a task for medical doctors. As decision makers, we can say that we need a length of time of about 35 years to develop courses at the European level in order to be informed – about eHealth, about other technologies, administrative regulations, data protection – in order to build integration of these points into the basic decision making process.

This is why, as I mentioned before, the open method of co-ordination with the member states could be one of the administrative instruments. The second administrative instrument we can put in place is the so-called international collaboration with a lot of technological platforms. Now we have the concept of a European eHealth area.

We have two instruments: the open method of co-ordination, essentially for policy makers, and the technical instrument of the technological platform. This instrument will be clearly described next May 2004 in Cork and a group will immediately be established to facilitate the implementation of eHealth.

As a part of the legal aspect, we have a lot of communalities in the domain of data protection, digital signature, consumer protection, guidance, documents, intellectual property rights etc. This document is new and it will be largely disseminated, in particular through EHTEL, if you agree.

But in addition, we can maybe document a guideline for implementation. In particular, a big issue that Canada shares a lot with the European Union is a thin layer of a federal approach with only small responsibility and strong implementation, set in place by the provinces (or member states or regional authorities). So the meta-structure is the same. With Canada, we share common views, common values, we respect data protection and have a multicultural, multilingual approach. This is not the case with the US. This is why we can easily exchange concepts and techniques with Canada. Recently, a national initiative for TeleHealth was drafted by the University of Calgary on behalf of the federal authority of Canada. This document is very, very beneficial and could be disseminated as well to all decision makers, through EHTEL, if you agree.

There are two other guidelines I mentioned before: the open method of co-ordination and the technological platform. As a part of the education process, the European Institute of Management for Public Services based in Maastricht will in September 2004 start a high level course concerning eHealth. It will be available one day a month for nine months and it will be restricted to a few, maximum 50, high level civil servants. I am sure these individual courses will be beneficial for facilitating the transfer of technology and implementation.

The financial soft spot, I mentioned before. But do you know where the bottleneck is at the moment? It is not the money; the bottleneck lies in the conservatism. It has been mentioned before referring to health care professionals, to patients and so on, but in particular it applies to the banks, the European Bank in Luxembourg, the World Bank in Washington, the European Bank for Reconstruction and Development in London. The banks cultivate a background concept of no risk. If Brazil or Venezuela make a request for aid in solving a problem, in re-engineering a system – if the World Bank supports a hospital, no risk. No politician can blame the banks. If the alternative proposition is based on eHealth, they doubt it; it is a risky approach. So it is urgent now to convince the World Bank authorities, the European Investment Bank and the European Bank for Reconstruction and Development to integrate eHealth solutions as part of their initiatives. If not, we will develop a lot of intelligent products and we will try to develop the best possible implementation plan, but we need the agreement from all banks. It will guide the change of implementation from traditional solutions which are outdated and not efficient at all. That is why it is urgent now to convince the international banks to integrate eHealth as a part of the game.

Another useful initiative is, as a result of the HINE report, a national plan for implementation. We have a survey highlighting what is the situation in Belgium, Italy, Germany, France and so on concerning the implementation of eHealth. What about the top ten already implemented – and what about the top next eHealth solution plans to be implemented in the next three years? It is once again a demonstration of the booming implementation of eHealth.

List of Authors

Ivo Burger, Municipal Hospital in Litomerice, Czech Republic

Dr. Gottfried Dietzel, Telematics – Health Card Project Group at the Federal Ministry of Health and Social Security, Germany

Prof. Dr. Jean-Claude Healy, European Commission, DG INFSO, Brussels

Ole Henriksen, European Commission, DG SANCO, Luxemburg

Mats Larson, Carelink, Sweden

Dr. José Luis Monteagudo, Ministry of Health and Consumption, Spain

Ákos Moró, Ministry of Health, Social and Family Affairs, Hungary

Norbert Paland, Telematics – Health Card Project Group at the Federal Ministry of Health and Social Security, Germany

Prof. Dr. Otto Rienhoff, Vice President of EHTEL

Angelo Rossi Mori, Institute for Biomedical Technology of the National Research Council, Italy

Marjan Suselj, Health Insurance Institute of Slovenia

Michèle Thonnet, President of EHTEL

Dr. Manfred Zipperer, Chairman of the Action Forum on Health Telematics, Germany

Prof. Dr. Jana Zvárová, EuroMISE Centre of Charles University and Academy of Sciences, Czech Republic

Organizing Committee

Katharina Bauch, ZTG Centre for Health Telematics

Dr. Gottfried Dietzel, Federal Ministry of Health and Social Security

Jürgen Dolle, Association for Social Security Policy and Research (GVG)

Dr. Erhard Geiss, Association for Social Security Policy and Research (GVG)

Dr. Frank Hackenberg, Association of Salaried Employees Sickness Funds, Association of Wage-Earners Sickness Funds

Franz Hertl, German Telecom AG

Anja Jansen, Association for Social Security Policy and Research (GVG)

Ute Lützenkirchen, Association for Social Security Policy and Research (GVG)

Reinhold Mainz, National Association of Statutory Health Insurance Physicians

Mathias Redders, Ministry of Health, Social Affairs, Women and Family of the State of North-Rhine/Westphalia

Dr. Kirsten Reinhard, AOK-BV – Federal Association of the General and Local Health Care Funds

Claudia Riepe, Federal Ministry of Health and Social Security

Regina Rösler, Saxony State Ministry of Social Affairs

Dr. Rainer Wedekind, Saxony State Ministry of Social Affairs

Dr. Manfred Zipperer, Action Forum on Health Telematics (ATG)

Programme Committee (virtual)

Hans-Peter Bursig, German electrical and electronic manufacturers' association (ZVEI)

Dr. Gottfried Dietzel, Federal Ministry of Health and Social Security

Jürgen Dolle, Association for Social Security Policy and Research (GVG)

Prof. Dr. Joachim W. Dudeck, Institute for Medical Informatics at the University of Giessen

Dr. Wolfgang Dierker, German Association for Information Technology, Telecommunications and New Media e. V. (BITKOM)

Dr. Erhard Geiss, Association for Social Security Policy and Research (GVG)

Dr. Jörg Haas, Top Association Information Technology in Health Care System

Prof. Dr. Peter Haas, German Association for Medical Informatics, Biometry and Epidemiology

Dr. Frank Hackenberg, Association of Salaried Employees Sickness Funds, Association of Wage-Earners Sickness Funds

Franz Hertl, German Telecom AG

Stephan Hoffmann, Siemens Medical Solutions

Reinhold Mainz, National Association of Statutory Health Insurance Physicians

Mathias Redders, Ministry of Health, Social Affairs, Women and Family of the State of North-Rhine/Westphalia

Prof. Dr. Helmut Reimer, TeleTrusT Deutschland e. V.

Dr. Kirsten Reinhard, AOK-BV – Federal Association of the General and Local Health Care Funds

Peter Reuschel, InterComponentWare AG

Prof. Dr. Otto Rienhoff, Clinical Data Processing Centre of the University Hospital Göttingen

Jürgen Sembritzki, ZTG Centre for Health Telematics

Dr. Rainer Wedekind, Saxony State Ministry of Social Affairs

Prof. Dr. Alfred Winter, German Association for Medical Informatics, Biometry and Epidemiology

Dr. Manfred Zipperer, Action Forum on Health Telematics (ATG)

Contact Address *eHealth 2003*

Gesellschaft für Versicherungswissenschaft und -gestaltung e. V.
ATG Aktionsforum Telematik im Gesundheitswesen
Hansaring 43
D-50670 Köln

Phone: ++49 (221) 912867-23
Fax: ++49 (221) 912867-6
Email: atg@gvg-koeln.de
Internet: http://atg.gvg-koeln.de

The Congress *eHealth 2003* was organized by:

Jürgen Dolle
Co-ordinator ATG, Cologne
Phone: ++49 (221) 912867-23
Email:j.dolle@gvg-koeln.de

Anja Jansen
ATG, Cologne
Phone: ++49 (221) 912867-21
Email: a.jansen@gvg-koeln.de

Sandy Lange
Assistant at the ATG, Cologne

Ute Lützenkirchen
ATG, Cologne
Phone: ++49 (221) 912867-19
Email: u.luetzenkirchen@gvg-koeln.de

Action Forum on Health Telematics (ATG)

The Action Forum on Health Telematics (ATG) joins the different actors in the German health care system at one table, it creates transparency and consensus opportunities and prepares recommendations which serve as an important orientation basis for all contracting parties in the health system and the responsible ministries. The goal of the ATG is to make use of telematics as an important tool for the further development of health care enhancing both the quality and the cost efficiency of care.

The ATG is dealing both with the technical-organisational infrastructure and the requirements of such infrastructure as regards concrete applications (e.g. electronic prescription, electronic referral and discharge letter and the international dimension of telematics applications, electronic health record, patient information systems, anonymisation / pseudonymisation) as well as with the general framework for the use of telematics in health care.

The ATG may contribute to the comprehensive co-operation of the different telematics initiatives at national level. The process of establishing a telematics platform for the German health care system is understood not only to be an organisational-technical procedure, but also to be a process of political opinion-forming, bundling all social actors concerned with this topic. The self-governing organisations in health care have come to control the process of designing telematics applications in health care through their active participation.

The organisations supporting the ATG aim to establish a common IT infrastructure, design joint applications or set a suitable framework. The goal is to optimise the quality of medical care and open up rationalisation potentials through the cross-sector use of information technology in selected fields of health care.

To this end, comprehensive agreements must be entered into, which reflect both the general framework and the technical-organisational basis for the use of interoperable solutions and, as a consequence, form the prerequisite for a sustainable improvement of workflows and the data situation of all parties involved.

Action recommendations on concrete nation-wide and comprehensive routine applications in the information and communication process of health care (electronic prescription, electronic referral and discharge letter) and on the establishment and operation of a generally valid communication and security infrastructure that is used by all parties involved can be used by the different self-governing organisations and by the government and politicians as decision-making aids for the first steps towards the jointly structured use of information and communication technology in health care.

The Action Forum on Health Telematics (ATG) is able to avoid a further divergence of emerging solutions by working out the optimum solutions with the people responsible in administrations, governments, industry and science, which are then fixed by the responsible bodies of the parties involved as jointly agreed procedures.

A long-term strategy will be discussed and determined upon common consensus. Among other things, the type of realisation of a cross-institutional treatment documentation (electronic patient record) as the future core element of a cross-sector co-operation must be dealt with during this process.

Publications

Gesellschaft für Versicherungswissenschaft und -gestaltung e.V. – GVG (Hrsg.): eHealth 2003 – Telematik im Gesundheitswesen: Vernetzte Versorgung. Dokumentation zum nationalen und internationalen Kongress, 21. bis 23. Oktober 2003 im Hilton Hotel Dresden. Köln 2004.

Gesellschaft für Versicherungswissenschaft und -gestaltung e.V. – GVG (Hrsg.): ATG-Forum, Telematik-Rahmenarchitektur für das Gesundheitswesen. Sitzung vom 16. Dezember 2002. Informationsdienst Nr. 289, Köln März 2003.

Gesellschaft für Versicherungswissenschaft und -gestaltung e.V. – GVG (Hrsg.): eHealth 2002 – Telematik im Gesundheitswesen. Dokumentation zum nationalen und internationalen Kongress, 5. bis 7. März 2002 im Maritim Hotel Bonn. Köln 2002.

Gesellschaft für Versicherungswissenschaft und -gestaltung e.V. – GVG (Hrsg.): Dr. Stephan H. Schug: Europäische und internationale Perspektiven von Telematik im Gesundheitswesen. Internationale Studie des Aktionsforums Telematik im Gesundheitswesen. Köln 2001.

Gesellschaft für Versicherungswissenschaft und -gestaltung e.V. – GVG (Hrsg.): Aktionsforum Telematik im Gesundheitswesen: Dokumentation zur zweiten Plenumsveranstaltung. Köln / Berlin 2001.

Gesellschaft für Versicherungswissenschaft und -gestaltung e.V. – GVG (Hrsg.): Aktionsforum Telematik im Gesundheitswesen: Erwartungen der Partner im Gesundheitswesen an eine moderne Infrastruktur. Köln / Baden Baden 2000.

For our **online publications** please visit our website: http://atg.gvg-koeln.de